Birth Defects and Speech-Language Disorders

Birth Defects and Speech-Language Disorders

Shirley N. Sparks, MS
Western Michigan University
Kalamazoo, MI

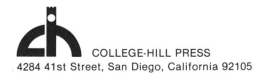

COLLEGE-HILL PRESS
4284 41st Street, San Diego, California 92105

College-Hill Press
4284 41st Street
San Diego, California 92105

Library of Congress Cataloging in Publication Data

Main entry under title:
Sparks, Shirley N. (Shirley Nichols),
    Birth defects and speech-language disorders

    Includes bibliographical references and index.
    1. Speech disorders in children — Genetic aspects.
2. Language disorders in children — Genetic aspects.
3. Abnormalities, Human — Complications and sequelae.
4. Fetus — Abnormalities — Complications and sequelae.
5. Handicapped children — Language. I. Title.
RJ496.S7S6 1984   618.92'855   83-23917
ISBN 0-933014-06-6

Printed in the United States of America

To my husband and our children
Steven, Ann, and John

Contents

Preface

"A birth defect is an abnormality of structure, function, or metabolism. It is genetically determined, or the result of environmental influence on the unborn child. In many cases, a combination of both may be the cause" (March of Dimes).

Speech-language clinicians* treat children who have genetic disorders and birth defects daily in schools, clinics, or institutions. In fact, the clinician may be the first professional to suspect the existence of a genetic or environmental birth defect. Birth defects have received much attention from the medical profession, but physicians' chief concerns are not speech and language. Consequently, descriptions of genetic disorders in the medical literature concentrate on physical features. There are a number of volumes devoted to the cataloging of syndromes and birth defects (Bergsma, 1979; McKusick, 1978; and Smith, 1982). These sources should not be overlooked for information on prognosis, progressive or nonprogressive disability, or mental retardation in a disorder. Bergsma lists "speech" in the index with items of delayed, indistinct, slow, scanning, and slurred speech in a total of 47 of the 1,005 syndromes cataloged in the volume. However, a clinician may research a disorder in one of these texts but not find definitive descriptions of speech and language.

The primary purpose of this book is to serve as a resource for signs and symptoms and for prognoses of birth defects for speech-language clinicians in clinical practice and for students. The *signs* are objective physical findings, while *symptoms* are subjective (personal descriptions by the patient of the experience or change due to the disorder). A discussion of fetal development, basic genetics, and some important underlying principles of biology are presented, not only to answer some questions, but to raise some questions of etiology of speech and language disorders. Most of the information considered basic to understanding genetics contained in Chapter 1 was not known 20 years ago. Therefore, clinicians with a knowledge of basic genetics may have more knowledge of the topic than physicians who graduated from medical school prior

---

* Speech-language pathology practitioners will be referred to hereafter as clinicians.

to 1960. Chapters 2 through 5 discuss the principles of chromosomal, single-gene, multifactorial, and environmental disorders that may affect speech and language. Birth defects that cause speech and language disorders occur in the perinatal as well as the prenatal period, and those disorders are discussed in Chapter 6, along with suggestions for the hospitalized child. Specific diagnostic and history-taking procedures are outlined in the appendices.

The second goal is to bring to the attention of clinicians (Chapter 7) a resource that is new on the clinical scene and is almost untapped by the profession of speech-language pathology: genetic counseling. Weitz (1981) notes that the use of genetic counseling may be restricted by a lack of knowledge on the part of both physicians and potential clients, by such social-psychological barriers as fear of genetic disease and its attendant stigma, by beliefs derived from the general culture and the medical culture, and by financial considerations. There is a critical need for public education about the prevention of genetic diseases and mental retardation (Milunsky, 1981). Only with an educated profession and public alike can the dramatic advances in medical genetics benefit all of us.

The final goal is to stimulate research by clinicians. Most of the studies cited here originated in other disciplines. IQ tests were used for the evaluation of verbal abilities instead of standardized speech and language tests. But there are some model studies. Witkop and Henry conducted research as early as 1963 that suggested that specific genetic inborn errors of metabolism were related to specific speech behaviors (Chapter 3). There are two obvious barriers to biochemical and genetic research by practicing clinicians: The language of genetics is foreign, and clinicians have little access to the laboratory sciences of genetics. Interdisciplinary investigations may be the answer for specific biochemical investigations. But clinicians can report individual case studies. Much of the speech and language information in the literature is composed of studies of single cases or of a small number of affected individuals similar to those included here. Single case studies are not meant to provide enough information to guide therapy for other children with the same condition. Furthermore, research in the area of prevention of prenatal environmental and multifactorial defects is crucial. In Chapter 8, some guidelines for effective research by clinicians are outlined.

The contents of this book have been drawn from my experience as a clinician and teacher in a university speech-language hearing clinic and as a member of the staff of a genetics clinic. I am indebted to several of my colleagues from the Kalamazoo Genetics Clinic at Western Michigan University for their help and reviews of the manuscript: Leonard Ginsberg, PhD, geneticist and biochemist; Donald Johnson, MD, pediatrician; and Gretchen Landenberger, MS, genetic counselor. I am grateful also to John Hanley, PhD, and Clyde Willis, PhD, speech pathologists at Western Michigan University, for review of the manuscript, and to former students Sidney Millard, Karen Zalewski, and Leslie Schmidt for research assistance. I particularly wish to acknowledge the invaluable guidance in preparation of the manuscript of Robert Erickson, PhD, chairman of the Department of Speech Language Pathology and Audiology at Western Michigan University. John Phillips, MD, of Tulane University College of Medicine, also provided technical assistance. Of special importance was the support, encouragement, and vigilance in perusing the medical literature of my physician husband, Robert D. Sparks, MD. I wish to give a special thanks to the children with whom I have been privileged to work and to their parents, who so willingly contributed pictures and personal stories.

REFERENCES

Bergsma, D. (Ed.) Birth defects compendium (2nd ed.). New York: Allan J. Liss, 1979.

March of Dimes. All about the March of Dimes. Brochure no. 9-0059. Jan., 1980.

McKusick, V.A. Mendelian inheritance in man (5th ed.). Baltimore: Johns Hopkins University Press, 1978.

Milunsky, A. Prenatal diagnosis of genetic disorders. American Journal of Medicine, 1981, 70, 7-8.

Smith, D.W. Recognizable patterns of human malformation (3rd ed.). Philadelphia: Saunders, 1982.

Weitz, R. The public, the primary physician and genetic counseling. First Quarter, 1981, 3, 13-16.

Witkop, C.J., & Henry, F.V. Sjogren-Larsson syndrome and histidinemia, hereditary biochemical diseases with defects of speech and oral functions. Journal of Speech and Hearing Disorders, 1963, 28, 109-123.

Introduction

In her excellent discussion of differential diagnosis of speech and language disturbances, Beadle (1981) describes the confusion for clinicians that revolves around the identification of underlying etiologies:

> The issue of causation is often avoided or dealt with only superficially. This may reflect the fact that the term "diagnosis" tends to be associated with a medical model, and speech and language pathologists cannot make medical diagnoses. Nevertheless, the individuals and families who consult professionals regarding speech and language disturbances want an answer to the question *WHY?* as well as to the question *WHAT?* From the standpoint of effective intervention, it is necessary to understand both the cause and the nature of a problem. (p.284)

Clinicians are accustomed to dealing with the behavioral aspects of their patients. In some disorders the physical aspects must be dealt with as well. A clinician would not be expected to give adequate therapy to an aphasic patient without first having a thorough understanding of stroke and the specific damage it can cause to the brain. A clinician treating a patient with cleft palate is expected to understand the anatomy of the head and how the palatal structures are joined during fetal development. From this knowledge of the cause, the clinician better understands the nature of the problem.

Speech and language disorders are steadily being subtracted from the large category called "functional" and added to the small but growing category of disorders with physical etiology. The relatively new field of cytogenetics, the branch of genetics that correlates changes in the number and arrangement of chromosomes with changes in the structure and function of organisms, has provided a breakthrough in the discovery of etiologies for many behavioral, as well as physical, disorders. In 1953, Watson and Crick described the structure of DNA, and advances in genetics have been rapid and exciting since that time. The clinical study of human chromosomes has been possible for only slightly less than 25 years. In 1956, investigators in Sweden systematically counted 46 chromosomes in human cells: 22 pairs and the sex chromosomes. Previously, the number of human chromosomes had been thought to be 48. Chromosome identification techniques were quickly applied to clinical medical practice. In 1959, researchers identified an extra chromosome 21 in patients with Down syndrome. Identification of other classic cytogenetic disorders, such as in what was previously thought to be nonspecific mental retardation, soon followed. Genetic carrier status could be determined for translocation in chromosomal disorders. The development of banding techniques for individual chromosomes was the next major breakthrough, which enabled researchers to recognize individual chromosomes and to detect subtle abnormalities within them (Bennett, 1981; Nyhan, 1983).

Although advances in genetic research have been explosive, new knowledge has grown unevenly. Much is known about birth defects due to single-gene mutations, but very little is known about environmentally-induced birth defects, those agents that act directly on the fetus or indirectly through the mother. Knowledge is scarce concerning additive effects involving multiple-gene causation of disease or defect. Almost nothing is known about the mechanisms of multifactorial (gene plus environment) defects (Ajl, 1982).

Until these discoveries occurred in the 1950s, American clinical medicine paid little attention to genetics. In fact, few American medical schools provided more than introductory instruction in genetics. But gradually, clinical genetics has been incorporated into the practice of medicine. In 1900, 1 infant death in approximately 25 was due to congenital malformation; now it is about 1 in 5 (Porter, 1979). Twenty to 30% of pediatric inpatients have diseases in which genetic factors appear to play a significant role (Summer & Shoaf, 1982). There is a striking difference between those physicians who graduated more than 10 years ago and more recent graduates in terms of their knowledge of genetics (Porter, 1979).

In the 1950s, when the discoveries were made in cytogenetics, speech pathology was in its early days. As speech pathology became speech-language pathology and the importance of cognitive damage to language learning became more apparent, physical medicine, particularly neurology, gained in importance. The profession of audiology has recognized the importance of genetic discoveries in otolaryngologic disorders (Konigsmark & Gorlin, 1976; Pashayan, 1973) and incorporated that knowledge into university academic programs. Speech-language pathology has traditionally been involved in the treatment of individuals with Down syndrome, cleft palate, and maxillofacial anomalies, but it has paid little attention to genetic causes of language and speech disorders.

The explanation for language learning as inborn or genetic, with the pattern of development in a predictable sequence, has been suggested by Chomsky (1968) and Lenneberg (1967, 1969). A syndrome is defined as a collection of signs and symptoms from one cause. Are there genetic speech and language abnormalities, as well as physical signs, in some syndromes? Current investigations have uncovered common speech and language signs and symptoms in individuals with genetic syndromes. For example, in Down syndrome it is known that the trisomy of chromosome 21 affects all cells and that there are predictable patterns of articulation and language learning. Children affected by fetal alcohol syndrome have permanent growth retardation and exhibit an inability to catch up mentally and physically with normal children but a pattern of language retardation is less clear. Some syndromes have mental retardation as a sign, some have dysarthria or cleft palate, and some have hearing loss. What are others?

According to McKusick (1975, p.263) clinical genetics "is involved in all parts of the triad of clinical practice: diagnosis, prognosis, and treatment...What is wrong (diagnosis); what is going to happen (prognosis); and what can be done about it (treatment)." The first step toward understanding the cause and nature of a problem is accurate diagnosis and assessment. The clinician needs to ask these questions: What are the physical features of this disorder? What are the cognitive strengths and weaknesses dictated by the syndrome that will guide my plans for therapy? If the family does not have a diagnosis, how can I help them obtain a diagnosis? Is a genetics clinic the correct referral? Second, What is the prognosis for progress? The Code of Ethics of the American Speech-Language Hearing Association advises members not to provide treatment unless there is a probability of success. Third, there are two ways to provide treatment with genetic disorders. The first one is genetic engineering: ways of changing genes or substituting the right gene for a wrong one. No one has yet been able to do this in humans, but it may be possible in the future. The second method is prenatal or postnatal treatment of the disorder through drugs, diet, transfusion, organ transplantation, replacement of enzymes, or surgical repair and reconstruction. To these must be added habilitation to improve the quality of life for the affected individual; it is in this phase of treatment of genetic defects that the clinician plays a vital role.

There have been some notable shifts in the incidence of specific disorders. Vaccines have sharply reduced the number of children born with mental retardation caused by rubella. Prenatal diagnosis may be cutting the incidence of Down syndrome and some genetic diseases that can be identified in carrier parents and in fetuses. This reduction is largely balanced by the increase in pregnant women who smoke (a cause of low birth weight) and by better neonatal care that can save the lives of high-risk babies but cannot prevent consequent brain damage or iatrogenic (treatment-induced) problems.

On the other hand, as treatment of people with genetic disorders becomes more and more effective, it is expected that the incidence of genetic defects will rise in the general population, thus requiring more and more therapeutic services. The more successful the treatment, the more likely the increase of the carrier population (Ajl, 1982). For example, a disorder for which clinicians participate in successful treatment is cleft lip and palate. With surgical techniques and speech therapy, this disorder is corrected. If the affected person reproduces, more children are born who are genetically at risk for clefting (Chapter 4). Craniofacial disorders, such as Crouzon syndrome (Chapter 2), are another example of genetic disorders in which treatment allows individuals to lead normal lives and to pass on their genes.

When we understand what causes a disorder (diagnosis), we are better able to predict what is likely to happen (prognosis) and what can be done about it (therapy). When clinicians are familiar with the genetic basis for an abnormality, they will better understand the natural course of the condition and provide optimal therapy.

REFERENCES

Ajl, S.J. Birth defects research: 1980 and after. *American Journal of Medicine,* 1982, 72, 119-126.

Beadle, K.R. Speech and language disturbances in childhood development. In J.K. Darby, Jr. (Ed.), *Speech evaluation in medicine.* New York: Grune & Stratton, 1981.

Bennett, J. A primer in human genetics. In K.I. Abroms & J.W. Bennett (Eds.), *Issues in genetics and exceptional children.* San Francisco: Jossey-Bass, 1981.

Chomsky, N. *Language and mind.* New York: Harcourt, Brace, Jovanovich, 1966.

Konigsmark, B.W., & Gorlin, R.J., *Genetic and metabolic deafness.* Philadelphia: Saunders, 1976.

Lenneberg, E. *Biological foundations for language.* New York: Wiley, 1967.

Lenneberg, E. On explaining language. *Science*, 1969, *164*, 635-643.

McKusick, V.A. The growth and development of human genetics as a clinical discipline. *American Journal of Genetics*, 1975, *27*, 261-273.

McKusick, V.A. *Mendelian inheritance in man (5th ed.)*. Baltimore: Johns Hopkins University Press, 1978.

Nyhan, W.L. Cytogenic diseases, *Clinical Symposia*, Ciba, West Caldwell, NJ, 1983, 35(1).

Pashayan, H. *Genetic considerations in hearing disorders. Proceedings of the Conference of Orofacial Anomalies: Clinical and Research Applications* (ASHA Reports No. 8; pp.132-156), August 1973.

Porter, I. Introduction. In W. Stockton, *Altered destinies*. Garden City, NY: Doubleday, 1979.

Summer, G.K., & Shoaf, C.R. Developments in genetic and metabolic screening. *Family and Community Health*, 1982, 4(4), 13-29.

1

Introduction to Genetics and Signs of Genetic Disorders

In the United States, 3 million live births occur each year, among which are 100,000 to 150,000 infants affected by some form of genetic disorder (Summer & Shoaf, 1982). Congenital malfunctions, single-gene disorders, chromosomal anomalies, or combinations of these are diagnosed in 30% of all pediatric hospital admissions, with an estimated cost in excess of $1 billion annually. Of those congenital disorders that usually involve the services of a clinician, 25 to 30% have obvious genetic transmission, for example, 33% of severe mental retardation (Stein & Susser, 1978), 25% of clefting (Bixler, 1981), and 25% of congenital deafness (Bergstrom, 1980). In this chapter the vocabulary of elementary genetics is introduced, and the bases of hereditary transmission of genetic disorders, physical signs of genetic disorders, and genetics of mental retardation are discussed.

Genetics is the scientific study of heredity. Genes are the discrete hereditary units transmitted from parents to their offspring. Genes are made up of DNA (deoxyribonucleic acid), a self-replicating molecule that makes copies of itself with remarkable fidelity. When a change in DNA occurs, the change is copied and passed on to the next generation of cells. In 1865 an Austrian monk, Gregor Mendel, discovered the principle by which these hereditary units pass from one generation to the next; it is now known as Mendel's law. The genetic makeup of an individual is the *genotype*. It is established at conception; thereafter, a complex interaction of genes and environment shapes the observable characteristics that comprise an individual's *phenotype*. *Proband* refers to the particular individual exhibiting a disorder (Bennett, 1981).

The basic building blocks of a living system are its *cells*. The nucleus of a cell is a spherical body that functions as the control center. Genes are located in the nucleus, on pairs of microscopic bodies called *chromosomes*. The 23 pairs of human chromosomes differ in size and shape as well as in the genes they contain. A standardized system for the classification of human chromosomes has been devised. In this system, 22 of the 23 pairs are termed *autosomes*. The largest autosomal pair is labeled 1, the next largest 2, and so on down the line to the smallest pair, which is labeled 22. The remaining pair of chromosomes is not numbered. These are the sex chromosomes, and they are labeled X and Y. Females have 2X chromosomes (XX), and males have 1 X and 1 Y chromosome (XY).

Human chromosomes can be studied conveniently if cells are grown in the laboratory from white blood cells, skin, or amniotic fluid and then treated and stained so that individual chromosomes can be seen under a microscope. A photograph of the chromosomes from a cell (a chromosome spread) is taken. The photograph is cut apart and the chromosomes are arranged by size and shape. The resulting arrangement of chromosomes is called a *karyotype* (Bennett, 1981).

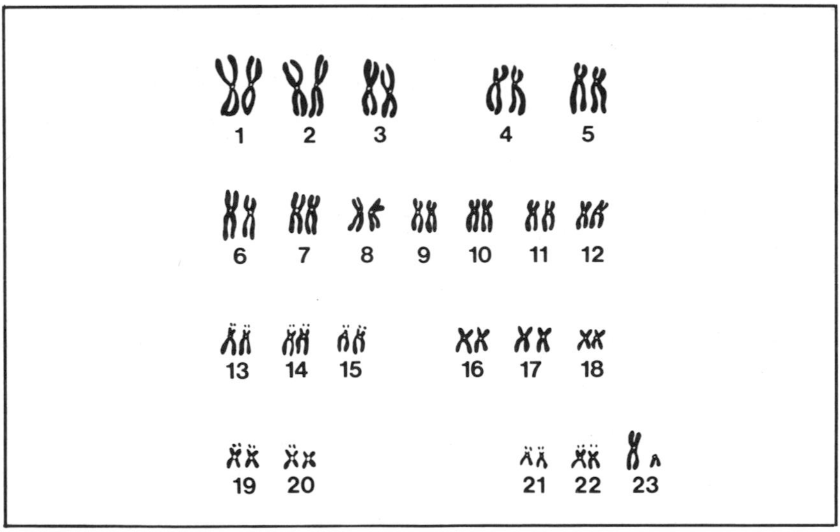

FIGURE 1-1
A karyotype of a normal male showing 22 pairs of autosomes and two sex chromosomes. From *Is My Baby Alright?* by V. Apgar & J. Beck, 1972, Trident Press, Copyright 1972 by Joan Beck. Reprinted by permission of Simon and Schuster.

The symbol p is given to the short arm and q to the long arm of a chromosome. A + or − placed before a chromosome number indicates addition or loss of a whole chromosome; for example, +21 indicates an extra chromosome, as in Down syndrome. Placed after the chromosome number, these symbols indicate increase or decrease in the length of a chromosome part; for example, $5p$ − indicates loss of a part of chromosome 5, as in cri du chat syndrome (Thompson & Thompson, 1980).

GENOTYPE

The exact number of genes present on any human chromosome is not known, but the total number of functioning genes in a cell is about 25,000. Each gene is located on a chromosome in a specific position called the *locus*. One member of each chromosome pair is inherited from the mother, the other from the father. Since chromosomes exist in pairs, genes at a particular locus also exist in pairs. The two genes that occupy the same locus are called *alleles*. If both genes are the same, the individual is said to be *homozygous* at that particular locus. If the two alleles are different, the individual is *heterozygous* at that locus (Bennett, 1981).

The three main categories of genetic disorders are: (a) single-gene disorders, which are inherited in recognizable patterns; (b) chromosomal disorders, which are alterations in the number of chromosomes or in the structure of a single chromosome; and (c) multifactorial disorders, in which many genes and environmental factors interact. The complexities of multifactorial disorders will be discussed in Chapter 4. The genotypes of chromosomal and single-gene disorders follow a more well-defined pattern (see Chapters 2 and 3).

SINGLE-GENE DISORDERS

Approximately 3,000 conditions have been identified as single-gene defects, and, for these, the risk of producing affected offspring can be predicted mathematically (McKusick, 1978). Risk of recurrence in single-gene disorders is expressed in terms of percentages; the same risk is present for each pregnancy. Single-gene disorders follow three basic patterns of inheritance: autosomal dominant; autosomal recessive; and sex linked. In each case, the distinctive pattern of inheritance describes the transmission of the abnormal allele of the gene rather than the normal allele. Each of these three patterns can be studied using the technique of *pedigree analysis*.

Pedigrees are diagrams of family histories in which males are designated by squares and females by circles. Probands are designated by solid squares or circles; unaffected individuals are shown by open squares or circles. Each generation is numbered with a Roman numeral, while individuals within a generation are given Arabic numerals. Matings are shown by a horizontal line between two individuals. A double horizontal line is used to represent mating between known relatives (consanguineous mating). Single children are shown by a vertical line from the mating line, while several children are drawn along an inverted T shape (Bennett, 1981).

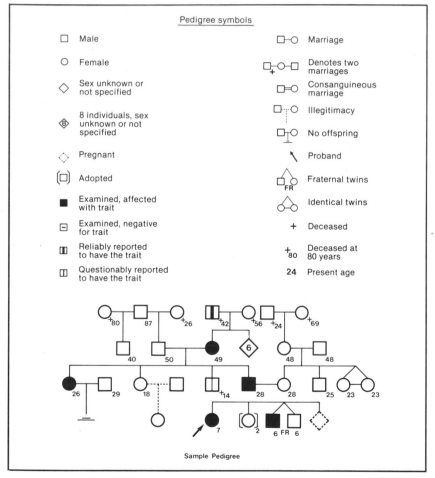

FIGURE 1-2
Pedigree symbols.

Expression and Penetrance

The concepts of expression and penetrance play an important part in the analysis of a pedigree for a trait. Within a single family, affected individuals may show a differing number of abnormalities, which make the disorder more or less severe, even though they are due to the same allele of the gene. The degree of severity is referred to as the *expressivity* of a trait. Thus, an individual with a syndrome may have one, more than one, or all signs of the disorder. For example, a person with Van der Woude syndrome may have lip pits, cleft of the hard palate, and bifid uvula, or he may have none of those expressions and still have the genotype for Van der Woude syndrome. *Penetrance* is whether or not a trait is expressed at all. If expressed, no matter how slightly, the gene is penetrant; if an individual has the gene but does not express it, it is *nonpenetrant*. Nonpenetrance results in an apparent skip in generations, and accounts for fewer than the expected number of children observed to be affected. Penetrance is an all-or-none concept. In mathematical terms, it is the percentage of genetically susceptible individuals who actually show a trait. When the frequency of expression of a trait is below 100%, that is, when an individual has the genotype but fails to express it, the trait is said to have *reduced penetrance*. For example, if only 80 out of every 100 persons carrying a single abnormal gene are affected, the gene is said to have 80% penetrance (Smith, D.W., 1982; Thompson & Thompson, 1980).

SINGLE-GENE TRANSMISSION

Autosomal Dominant Inheritance

When only one abnormal gene in a pair causes the abnormal condition, that is, when it is inherited from only one parent, and the gene is located on an autosome, the trait is inherited as an autosomal dominant. The following rules of transmission apply (Pernoll, King, & Prescott, 1980):

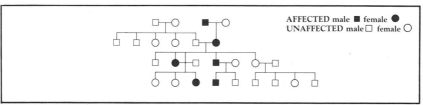

FIGURE 1-3
Autosomal dominant inheritance. The trait appears in each generation.

1. The trait can appear in each generation without skipping. Every affected person has at least one affected parent.

2. An affected person mating with a nonaffected person has, on the average, an equal number of affected and nonaffected children (occurrence is 50% regardless of the outcome of previous pregnancies).

3. Nonaffected children of affected parent(s) have nonaffected children and grandchildren.

4. Males and females are affected in equal numbers.

5. The affected person can be assumed to be a heterozygote (having only one abnormal allele for this gene).

New mutations

Permanent, heritable changes in DNA may arise spontaneously in any generation. An autosomal dominant pedigree must begin with a mutation, a common event in autosomal dominant disorders. For example, in Crouzon syndrome, most cases have no family history of the disorder and would thus presumably represent new mutations. However, all the affected individuals would be capable of transmitting the newly mutated genes to their own offspring.

Homozygous dominant genotype

Two alleles can only occur in the offspring of two individuals who each transmit the same dominant gene. In the known matings between persons with the same autosomal dominant disorder, such as achondroplastic dwarfs, the numbers of spontaneous abortions and stillborn infants with multiple malformations are increased, suggesting that a pair of dominant alleles may have a synergistic effect that is incompatible with survival.

Autosomal Recessive Inheritance

This category of transmission refers to autosomal genes that require abnormal genes on both alleles to be expressed, or one from each parent. The affected individual is said to have a homozygous recessive genotype. Recessive traits are expressed only in homozygotes and are hidden in heterozygotes. Heterozygous individuals who are phenotypically normal but carry a masked recessive gene, are called *carriers*; in some instances they can be identified by a laboratory screening test, for example, Tay-Sachs disease, sickle-cell anemia, and phenylketonuria (PKU) (see Chapter 7). The rules of transmission are (Pernoll et al., 1980):

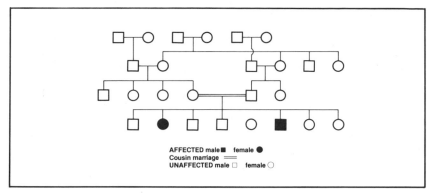

FIGURE 1-4
Autosomal recessive inheritance. Unaffected parents have affected children.

1. If an affected person is born to normal parents, both parents are heterozygotes (carriers), and there is a 25% chance that the normal parents' offspring will be affected, a 50% chance that they will be carriers, and a 25% chance that they will be normal (homozygous for the normal allele).

2. If an affected person mates with a genotypically normal person, all the children will be phenotypically normal heterozygotes.

3. If an affected person mates with a heterozygote, an average of one half of their children will be affected, and one half will be unaffected heterozygotes.

4. If two affected people mate, all of their children will be affected.

5. If a heterozygote mates with a person who produces a new mutation for that trait, it can result in an autosomal recessive trait.

6. Males and females are equally likely to be affected.

Most autosomal recessive disorders are rare in general populations but include the majority of inborn errors of metabolism (see Chapter 3). Although two out of three of the phenotypically normal siblings of an affected person are heterozygotes, their chance of mating with a carrier of the same mutant gene is remote because the conditions are uncommon. Therefore, the chance of having affected offspring is even more remote. Consanguineous mating (between blood relatives), increases the chances of having affected children due to the increased likelihood of carriers for a recessive disorder existing within the same family.

X-Linked Inheritance

A different pattern of inheritance occurs when the abnormal gene is located on the X chromosome. The Y chromosome contains very few genes and, therefore, is not known to transmit disorders. However, some 200 disorders can be transmitted by mutant genes on the X chromosome (McKusick, 1978). Because a male has only one X chromosome, any defective gene on that chromosome, recessive or dominant, will produce the defective trait in the male. A female, who has two X chromosomes, usually has a normal gene on one X chromosome to counter an abnormal recessive gene on the other X chromosome. She would then be a carrier of the disorder but would not express it herself. None of the male offspring of a father with an X-linked disorder can inherit the disorder from him, because he transmits only his Y chromosome to his sons. None of the father's daughters will have the disorder either, but all of the daughters will be carriers. For a woman to be affected, she must be homozygous for the mutant allele; that is, it must be present in both of her X chromosomes. This can happen only if her father is affected and her mother is either heterozygous or homozygous for the mutant allele. Since most X-linked mutants are rare or are not able to reproduce, affected women are extremely rare. On occasion, women known to be heterozygous for X-linked mutations show varying degrees of clinical expression, but rarely as severely as an affected male. This is explained by atypical *lyonization* of the X chromosomes in which the X chromosome carrying the normal gene becomes inactive, while the X chromosome carrying the abnormal gene is left active (Thompson & Thompson, 1980). The following rules of transmission for X-linked inheritance apply (Bennett, 1981):

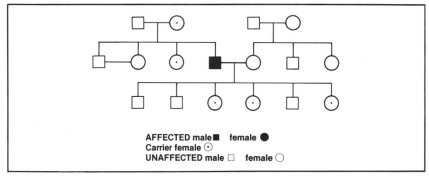

AFFECTED male ■   female ●
Carrier female ⊙
UNAFFECTED male □   female ○

FIGURE 1-5
X-Linked recessive inheritance. Females are carriers and males are affected.

1. Father-to-son inheritance is never observed. An affected father and a homozygous normal mother have all normal children; however, all the daughters are carriers.

2. A carrier female transmits the trait to one half of her sons; one half of her daughters become carriers.

3. More males than females express the trait.

4. The trait appears to skip generations, passing from affected fathers through unaffected carrier daughters and granddaughters to affected grandsons and great grandsons.

CHROMOSOMAL DISORDERS

Genetic disorders may be caused by a defect in an entire chromosome. The defect is not due to a single mistake in the genetic blueprint, but to an excess or deficiency of whole chromosomes or chromosome segments (Thompson & Thompson, 1980).

Translocation

Rarely, chromosomes are broken and rearranged. Most of the genes of the broken chromosome can then attach to another chromosome. The new chain of genes is called a *translocation chromosome*. A *balanced translocation carrier* is a person with a normal phenotype who has a translocation chromosome with the normal number of genes. The karyotype for a translocation denotes the increase or decrease in the length of that chromosome part (Thompson & Thompson, 1980).

Trisomy

Once an egg is fertilized, all further body cells are derived by the process of mitosis in which the newly combined chromosomes are divided equally into two daughter cells. One of the two chromosome pairs goes into each of the two new cells. If the chromosome duplicates do not properly separate, it is called *chromosome nondisjunction*. One of the new cells will have only one copy of the chromosome pair; a cell missing one chromosome usually does not develop further. The other new cell will have three copies of the chromosome, or a trisomy. All further cells with trisomy will have abnormal development. It is possible to have a trisomy of any chromosome. Sex chromosome trisomies can occur in a number of combinations from 47, XXX to 47, XYY (Thompson & Thompson, 1980). If the extra genetic material was a number 21 chromosome, a trisomy 21, or Down syndrome child is born. Of the autosomal trisomies, only 21, 13, and 18 usually produce live-born fetuses. It has been estimated that for every infant born with Down syndrome, two Down syndrome fetuses are spontaneously aborted. Approximately 95% of the conceptions of trisomies 8, 13, and 18 fail to survive the pregnancy (Hanson, 1977).

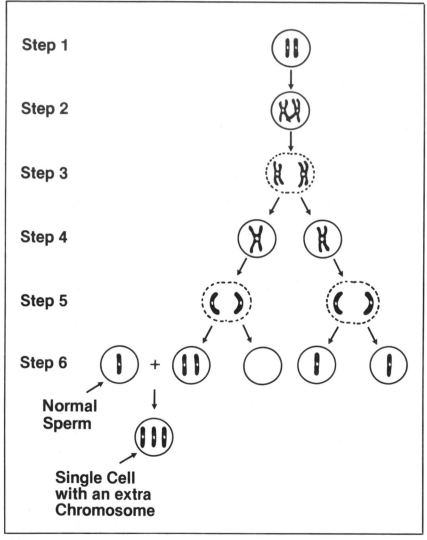

FIGURE 1-6
Trisomy nondisjunction. Down's Syndrome Congress, 1640 West Roosevelt Rd., Chicago, IL 60608. Reprinted by permission.

The risk for having a child with Down syndrome becomes greater each year after a woman is 35 years old (see Figure 1-7). In fewer than 5% of the cases, in the figure, one of the parents was a translocation carrier, but in the remainder, the cause is presumed

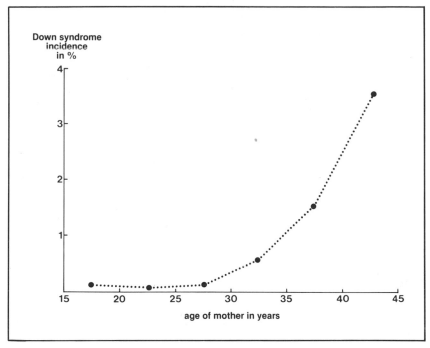

FIGURE 1-7
Incidence of Down syndrome with maternal age. From Down Syndrome brochure, Down's Syndrome Congress, 1640 West Roosevelt Rd., Chicago, IL 60608. Reprinted by permission.

to be a nondisjunction trisomy. The link of Down syndrome to advanced age of the mother seems plausible because of the difference in production of reproductive cells in males and females. Males do not produce sperm cells until they reach puberty, and, once begun, new production goes on continuously. However, the ovaries begin producing egg cells before a female is born. A baby girl is born with all the eggs she will ever produce stored within her body. The eggs are subjected to environmental insult throughout life, which may lead to increased nondisjunction in older women. However, with advances in cytogenetics, it has become apparent that advanced paternal age also carries an increased risk of chromosomal nondisjunction. Paternal origin may be responsible in one third of trisomic individuals (Abroms & Bennett, 1981; Ginsberg, L., personal communication, March, 1983; Nyhan, 1983). It should be noted also that male and female nondisjunction can occur at any age. Almost an equal number of Down syndrome children are born to women less than 30 years old as are born to women over 35.

Mosaic Trisomy

When a mitotic nondisjunction occurs in an embryo composed of only a few cells, further development results in a mix of normal cells and abnormal trisomy cells. Such a person is a chromosomal *mosaic*, or mixture of two different cell types. This person will have variable expression of the trisomy condition depending on the location (brain, liver, etc.) of the trisomic cells (Hanson, 1977).

PHENOTYPE

The phenotype is the entire physical, biochemical, and physiological nature of an individual as determined by his genotype and his environment (Thompson & Thompson, 1980). The language of hereditary disorders has etymological origins in Greek and Latin words concerning descent, birth, and origins. The combination of some of these terms provides a basic vocabulary for the description of disorders in the phenotype. *Morphology* is the branch of biology that deals with the structure and form of the organism at any stage of life. Thus, *dysmorphology* is impaired or abnormal structure. *Genesis* means the origin, creation, or beginning. *Morphogenesis* refers to the creation of the form, including growth and differentiation of cells and tissues during development. There are three basic types of anomalies (Smith, 1982): (a) A *malformation* is a structural defect that results from a localized abnormal development in morphogenesis. Cleft lip or palate caused by a single mutant gene is such a malformation. (b) A *deformation*, on the other hand, is an alteration in the structure or shape of a previously normally formed part due to mechanical factors. (c) A *disruption* is a primary malformation that causes other subsequent structural changes. Pierre Robin anomalad is an example of a disruption, because the characteristic cleft palate is actually incomplete closure of the palate secondary to the posterior displacement of the tongue, so that the palatal shelves must grow over the tongue to meet in the midline. A *syndrome* is a recognized pattern of malformations, presumably with the same cause. If a particular phenotype can be produced by a number of different genotypes, the phenotype is said to be *heterogeneous*. Pierre Robin anomalad is also an example of heterogeneity. It is most commonly seen in genotypically normal individuals, but it may also be a sign in sydromes with genetic etiology (Smith, D.W., 1982). Congenital deafness is another example of heterogeneity because it can be caused by several different genotypes.

Physical Signs of Dysmorphology

Not many years ago, all babies who weighed less than 5 pounds at birth were classified as premature. It is now known that there is more than one reason for low birth weight. The *premature* baby is an infant that is the expected size for its fetal age. The *small-for-gestational-age* infant is born on time but did not grow properly in utero. The latter category can be further divided into *primary* and *secondary* growth deficiency (Smith, D.W., 1982). Primary growth deficiency includes chromosomal and genetic disorders and inborn errors of metabolism. The growth failure is intrinsic to the fetus. In secondary growth deficiency, the fetus is affected by its environment, and, although the genetic coding is normal, the growth deficiency is secondary to a problem outside the fetus that limits its capacity for growth: delivery of nutrients, hormones, or oxygen to the cells. Secondary growth deficiency will be discussed in Chapter 5. This section will discuss the dysmorphologies of primary growth deficiency.

Some of the more common disorders, such as Down syndrome, are easily recognized, but every clinician has been confronted with children who have some nonspecific features of dysmorphology. Fifteen percent of the general population has a minor anomaly. Three minor anomalies or a major anomaly with many minor anomalies are found in 3% of the population. The incidence of major and/or minor anomalies may be higher among children with speech, language, or hearing impairments than in the population in general. Siegel-Sadewitz and Shprintzen (1980) found that 71% of a group of 42 speech-hearing, and learning-impaired children had at least one major malformation or two or more minor malformations. Although the children had a wide range of communication disorders, the most frequent anomalies found were dysmorphic eyes and ears and cranial malformations; these areas of the body are most complex and variable between individuals. The important considerations for the clinician to determine in a particular child suspected of exhibiting dysmorphology are (a) the *pattern of anomalies*, and (b) *overall growth retardation*, which constitutes an increased susceptibility to congenital malformations

(Spiers, 1982). If more than one of the following signs appear, there has been some dysmorphology (Smith, D.W., 1982):

1. Epicanthic folds of the eyes: A prominent fold of skin in the inner corner of the eye. Minor folds are normal and frequent in early infancy but disappear as the nasal bridge develops. (See Figure 1-8.)

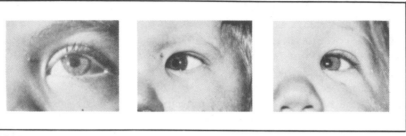

FIGURE 1-8
Inner epicanthic folds. From *Recognizable Patterns of Human Malformation* 3rd ed. by D.W. Smith, 1982, W.B. Saunders. Reprinted by permission.

2. Hypertelorism: Wide spacing of the eyes.

3. Ears low set or rotated: This represents a lag in body formation, since the ear is low and rotated in early fetal life. (See Figure 1-9.)

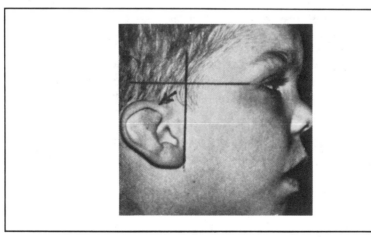

FIGURE 1-9
Ears are low set when the helix meets the cranium (arrow) at a level below that of a horizontal plane with the corner of the orbit. Ears are slanted when the angle of the slope of the auricle exceeds 15° from the perpendicular. From *Recognizable Patterns of Human Malformation* 3rd ed. by D.W. Smith, 1982, W.B. Saunders. Reprinted by permission.

4. Preauricular tags or pits just anterior to the ear. (See Figure 1-10.)

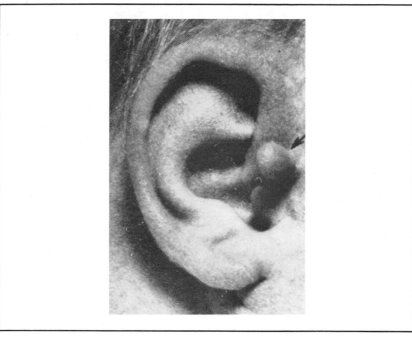

FIGURE 1-10
Preauricular tags, which often contain a core of cartilage. From *Recognizable Patterns of Human Malformation* 3rd ed. by D.W. Smith, 1982, W.B. Saunders. Reprinted by permission.

5. Genitalia unusually formed or small.

6. Unusual hair distribution: Very low hairline and heavy eyebrow growth denote abnormal growth in the upper face; unusual hair whorls; hirsutism.

7. Simian palm creases: Hand creases are formed by 11 weeks as the result of flexion of the hands by the fetus. Four percent of normal babies have simian creases. (See Figure 1-11.)

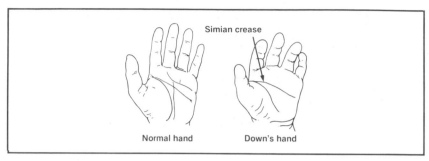

FIGURE 1-11
Hand of a child with Down syndrome has short, stubby fingers and a simian crease. From *Is My Baby Alright?* by V. Apgar and J. Beck, 1972, Trident Press, Copyright 1972 by Joan Beck. Reprinted by permission of Simon and Schuster.

    8. Curving fingers; stiff joints.
    9. Webbing of feet and hands.
  10. Absence of fingernails.
  11. Wide space between the first toe and others.
  12. Hypotonia of all muscles.
  13. Prominent lateral ridges on the palate.(See Figure 1-12.

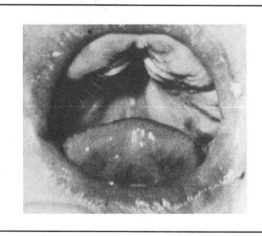

FIGURE 1-12
Prominent lateral palatal ridges may be a sign in a variety of disorders, especially those with serious neurologic deficits relative to sucking. From *Recognizable Patterns of Human Malformation* 3rd ed. by D.W. Smith, 1982, W.B. Saunders. Reprinted by permission.

14. Malproportion of the body.
15. Asymmetry, especially in the face.
16. Postnatal growth at a consistently slow pace.
(Growth charts, evaluation and referral procedures for the child with dysmorphology are provided in the appendices.)

Summary

Signs of dysmorphology in a child should alert the clinician to the possibility of a genetic disorder. Such signs are more likely to occur in a representative case load of speech-language- and hearing-impaired children than in the general population. The clinician should be alert to a pattern of anomalies exhibited, especially in the most complex areas of the body, and to evidence of overall growth deficiency. The clinician should pursue the possibility of a genetic disorder with a thorough case history and evaluation in order to make the proper referral for positive diagnosis. The diagnosis will dictate the guidelines for therapy: the physical features of the disorder, the communicative behaviors that are directly associated with the disorder and are presumably irreversible, the communicative behaviors that are amenable to change, and the prognosis for improvement.

GENETICS OF MENTAL RETARDATION

As we have seen in the previous section, the language of genetics is used to describe entities in a precise way. However, the vocabulary used to describe the condition of mental retardation is diverse, and mental retardation can only be arbitrarily defined. In general, mental retardation implies a condition in which an individual does not function intellectually according to societal definitions of normal. For the most part, intellectual normalcy becomes defined by certain standardized intelligence tests, which have language bases in varying degrees. For purposes of genetic description, an intelligence quotient (IQ) of below 50 will denote severe mental retardation and the mildy retarded will be in the group of those with IQ scores from 50 to 90.

Bearing this distinction in mind, it is possible to classify the genotypes of some mental retardation phenotypes. Mild mental retardation is approximately 3 to 10 times more common than severe mental retardation, and estimates of mild retardation vary widely according to sociocultural and economic family backgrounds. Only a small percentage of those with mild retardation have a chromosomal defect (Smith, G.F., 1981). The exceptions, however, are those with extra sex chromosomes, those with chromosome deletions, or those individuals who are mosaic. The severely retarded have more dysmorphologies and physical abnormalities than the mildly retarded, such as growth retardation, reduced head circumference, brain deformities, seizures, and spasticity. The association of three or more congenital anomalies with mental retardation suggests that disturbed brain function is due to a congenital anomaly (Smith, D.W.).

Genetic Mendelian traits account for 21 to 35% of all individuals with severe mental deficiency. The dominant traits account for 5% of the cases; recessive traits, 9%; and X-linked traits, 8% (Stein & Susser, 1978).

Severe retardation due to dominant traits is kept alive by the new mutation rate. Severe mental deficiency is associated with low reproductive rate, and in those with IQ below 25 there is almost complete absence of reproduction (Smith, G.F., 1981). Recessive traits account for many progressive disorders of severe mental deficiency. The disorders in this group range from severe physical abnormalities to inborn errors of metabolism. The exact cause of mental retardation in recessive disorders is usually quite specifically related to blocks in a biochemical pathway. A defect in any one of the multitude of steps and biochemical events involved in brain development may lead to a corresponding severe loss of mentation (Ginsberg, L., personal communication, March, 1983). (See Chapter 3.)

There are 32 known loci on the X chromosome that can produce both severe and mild mental retardation (McKusick, 1978) and more are reported continuously. All males who inherit the gene express it. The recently discovered fragile X chromosome syndrome is second only to Down syndrome as a genetic cause of mental retardation (Nyhan, 1983).

Mild mental retardation without physical abnormalities is the type found frequently in families. The etiology is thought to be multifactorial, an interaction of genetic susceptibility acting with environmental factors. There is approximately a 40% retardation rate in the children of a mating of two mildly retarded individuals. The risk factor is halved (20%) if one of the parents has normal intelligence (Smith, G.F., 1981).

Summary

The statement that the etiology of mental retardation is heterogeneous is not new in the field of speech-language pathology. However, clinicians who are well aware that the causes of retardation vary in their patients tend to lump these patients together under the heading "mentally retarded." Clinicians may ask what difference it makes in therapy if the etiology is chromosomal, Mendelian, or multifactorial, with or without physical abnormality.

Adler (1976) wrote that mentally retarded children possess a high incidence of speech defects characterized by articulation disorders, rhythm defects, expressive and receptive language disorders, and hearing impairments. He further noted that retarded children are not alike:

> Specifically, the incidence of oral communicative deficits in retardates vary in type and severity as a function of four interactive factors: (1) clinical genetic syndrome which in turn may affect (2) the structure and function of the oral and associated anatomy possessed by the child, as well as, (3) the severity of the retardation, which is also related to (4) the psychosocial environment in which the child is reared. Of particular importance, therefore, may be the child's genetic syndrome which influences all other factors. (p.136)

He warned that clinicians should desist from labeling a particular speech or language pattern as being common to all the retarded.

The etiology of an individual's mental retardation is of utmost importance for identification of those communication behaviors that are amenable to change and for prognosis. Mental retardation in chromosomal disorders is usually severe and is accompanied by physical features. On the other hand, the course of mental retardation as a result of a recessive metabolic disorder may become progressively worse, and the course of therapy is obviously quite different than in stable conditions. Mild mental retardation without physical abnormalities that is familial does not present the same clinical picture as mild mental retardation that is one of the signs of a syndrome. Diagnosis is the first step in the triad of clinical practice that leads to prognosis and treatment. The need for research to define those four interactive factors described by Adler cannot be overemphasized.

REFERENCES

Abroms, K.I., & Bennett, J.W. Parental contributions to trisomy 21. Review of recent cytological and statistical findings. In P. Mittler (Ed.), *Frontiers of knowledge in mental retardation. Vol. 2: Biomedical aspects.* Baltimore: University Park Press, 1981.

Adler, S. The influence of genetic syndromes upon oral communication. *Journal of Speech and Hearing Disorders,* 1976, *41,* 136-138.

Bennett, J.W. A primer in human genetics. In K.I. Abroms & J.W. Bennett (Eds.), *Issues in genetics and exceptional children.* San Francisco: Jossey-Bass, 1981.

Bergstrom, L. Causes of severe hearing loss in early childhood. *Pediatric Annals,* 1980, 9, 23-27.

Bixler, D. Genetics and clefting. *Cleft Palate Journal,* 1981, *18*(1), 10-18.

Hanson, M.J. *Teaching your Down's syndrome infant: A guide for parents.* Baltimore: University Park Press, 1977.

McKusick, V. *Mendelian inheritance in man* (5th ed.). Baltimore: Johns Hopkins Press, 1978.

Nyhan, W.L. Cytogenetic diseases. *Clinical Symposia,* Ciba, West Caldwell, NJ: 1983, 35(1).

Pernoll, M.L., King, C.R., & Prescott, G.H. Genetics for the obstetrician-gynecologist. *Obstetrics and Gynecology Annual,* 1980, 9, 1-53.

Siegel-Sadewitz, V.L., & Shprintzen, R.J. Major and minor malformations in a speech, hearing and learning impaired population. *Journal of New Jersey Speech and Hearing Association,* 1980, *17,* 17-21.

Smith, D.W. *Recognizable patterns of human malformation, genetic embryologic and clinical aspects* (3rd ed.). Philadelphia: Saunders, 1982.

Smith, D.W., & Bostian, K.E. Congenital anomalies associated with ideopathic mental retardation. *Journal of Pediatrics,* 1964, *65,* 189.

Smith, G.F. Genetics of mental retardation. In K.I. Abroms & J.W. Bennett (Eds.), *Issues in genetics and exceptional children.* San Francisco: Jossey-Bass, 1981.

Spiers, P.S. Does growth retardation predispose the fetus to congenital malformation? *Lancet,* 1982, 2, 312-314.

Stein, Z., & Susser, M. Epidemiologic and genetic issues. In N.E. Morton & L.S., Cheing (Eds.), *Mental retardation in genetic epidemiology.* New York: Academic Press, 1978.

Summer, G.K., & Shoaf, C.R. Developments in genetic and metabolic screening. *Family and Community Health,* 1982, 4, 13-29.

Thompson, J.S., & Thompson, M.W. *Genetics in medicine.* Philadelphia: Saunders, 1980.

2
Chromosomal Disorders

The incidence of chromosomal errors in live-born infants is approximately 1 in 200. It has been estimated that 1 in 13 conceptions has some kind of chromosomal aberration. About 15% of known pregnancies end in miscarriage; of these, approximately one half are chromosomally abnormal (Thompson & Thompson, 1980).

AUTOSOMAL CHROMOSOME SYNDROMES

The trisomies, translocations, and disjunctions that involve large pieces of genetic coding material necessarily involve the thousands of genes that are contained on that chromosome. Primary growth deficiency exhibited by retardation of development and multiple dysmorphic features are common to all autosomal aberrations regardless of which chromosome is involved and whether there is an excess or deletion of chromosomal material; the structures for speech and hearing and the cognition necessary for language will almost certainly be affected.

Down Syndrome

Down syndrome is caused by an excess of normal genetic material on chromosome 21 (see Chapter 1). It occurs in one of every 600 to 800 live births, and is the most common chromosomal anomaly (Nyhan, 1983). Mental retardation is almost universal, although differing degrees are seen in different individuals. It has been estimated that the majority of Down syndrome children fall in the IQ range of 30 to 50 (Kirk & Gallagher, 1979; Robinson & Robinson, 1976), but previous norms for IQ as well as language development were calculated on institutionalized Down syndrome children. Information on mental and language development has undergone radical change in the last few years because more Down syndrome children have been kept with their families and received early intervention and infant stimulation. Down syndrome has received particular attention from researchers in the last decade. A number of studies that have implications for speech and language therapy for Down syndrome have been conducted in medicine, occupational therapy, linguistics, and speech pathology.

Physical features in Down syndrome

Some of the general physical features of children with Down syndrome include: the back of the head is often flattened; the eyes are slanted upward; epicanthic folds are present at the inner corners of the eyes; the nasal bridge is slightly depressed; and the nose and ears are usually somewhat small. In the newborn there is often an excess of skin at the back of the neck. The hands and feet are small, and the fingerprint patterns are often different from the normal child's. The children have low muscle tone (hypotonia) causing hyperextension of joints (double jointedness). Children with Down syndrome remain small, and their physical and mental development is slow. Walking usually develops between 18 to 36 months (D.W. Smith, 1982; Stoel-Gammon, 1981).

Other congenital defects may be present in the Down syndrome child. About one third of these children have heart defects. The anatomical structure of the auditory system is more likely to be impaired than the structure of the visual system (Coleman, Schwartz, & Schwartz, 1979). An increased incidence of infection, particularly of the respiratory tract, occurs in Down syndrome. These children are particularly susceptible to middle ear infections, and examinations for otitis media should be performed frequently. Down syndrome is also associated with increased prevalence of such disease conditions as leukemia and other hematologic disorders, abnormalities of hypothalamic, pituitary, and adrenocortical function, and diabetes (Burch & Milunsky, 1969; Rowley, 1981). The prevalence of one common disease is decreased in Down syndrome: autopsy studies report virtual absence of atherosclerosis in older persons with Down syndrome, although they do experience premature aging. A progressive dementia develops that clinically resembles Alzheimer's disease (Heston, 1977). Persons with Down syndrome who survive into the later decades of life tend to die younger than other mentally handicapped persons of similar intelligence. Scoggin and Patterson (1982) conclude that the increased prevalence of leukemia, infection, endocrine dysfunction, and premature aging and the decreased incidence of atherosclerosis are influenced by the abnormal chromosome 21.

Speech and Language in Down Syndrome

Some anatomical differences specifically affect the speech structures (Stoel-Gammon, 1981): (a) an unusually high larynx and a short, unusually broad neck; (b) the presence of small, blunt styloid processes and deviations of other facial bones; (c) a high palate, shortness of the buccal cavity, and obstruction of the nasal passage; (d) an unusually small oral cavity, which gives the impression that the tongue is too large for the mouth.

It is possible that anatomical differences could account for some articulation problems as well as the low-pitched and hoarse voices prevalent in these children. Ardran, Harker, and Kemp (1972) found that protrusion of the tongue does not seem to be due to its enlargement but to the small jaw. The open mouth posture is often necessary to provide an airway, particularly if tonsils and adenoids are enlarged. The clinician who wishes to correct protrusion of the tongue should make sure that the child can breathe when the tongue is not extended.

Prelinguistic communication development

While the prelinguistic stages of development are similar to those of normal children, there are some striking differences. Lenneberg, Nichols, and Rosenberger (1964) followed the linguistic development of 61 noninstitutionalized Down syndrome children over a period of 3 years. They concluded that the development of the central nervous system is as crucial to language acquisition as it is to motor development. Therefore, attainment of motor milestones is as important a predictor of future language development as attainment of scores on standardized measurements of intelligence.

Jones (1980) looked at mother-infant interactions of six Down syndrome and normal infants and found few differences between the matched pairs in the frequency, length, variety, and channel (vocal or nonvocal) of the interactions. It was the way the children used their vocalizations that differed. The Down syndrome children tended to repeat sounds in strings, for example, "da, da, da," in contrast to the normal children's varied vocalizations, "da, ga, du." To these variations, the mothers of the normal children responded with rich and varied dialogue. The Down syndrome children's vocalizations were more repetitive and closer together than those of normal children, which did not allow a dialogue with their mothers. The mothers of the Down syndrome children simply acknowledged the child's vocalizations.

Jones (1980) also found that the Down syndrome children differed from normal children in their use of eye contact with their mothers. They did not avoid eye contact but simply failed to use the referential eye contact with their mothers that the normal children used. The normal children typically paused in their play and looked up at their mothers, and the mothers characteristically responded to this look by commenting about the previous play. The glance from the child seemed to be interpreted by the mothers as a questioning look and they responded with an answer.

Stoel-Gammon (1981) reviewed studies of prelinguistic utterances in Down syndrome (Dodd, 1975; B.L. Smith, 1977; B.L. Smith & Oller, 1981). The studies are similar in concluding that there is little or no difference, either qualitative or quantitative, between the vocalizations of normal and Down syndrome infants in the 1st year of life. During the 2nd year, however, a major difference appears. Among normally developing children, the first adultlike words typically appear around 13 to 15 months, at about the time the child also learns to walk. Among Down syndrome children, the onset of meaningful speech is later, and the rate of speech development is considerably slower. D.W. Smith and Wilson (1973) report that most Down syndrome children raised at home produce their first words between 2 and 3 years of age, although some children begin to talk soon after their first birthday and others not until the age of 7 or 8.

Early intervention in the prelinguistic stage

Some guidelines for therapy can be drawn from the preceding research into the relationship of linguistic development and central nervous system development. Furthermore, the hypotonia and floppiness of the Down syndrome child present problems for speech musculature as well as for all motor development. A promising method for early intervention is an interdisciplinary approach by a speech-language clinician and an occupational therapist using neurodevelopmental techniques. These techniques facilitate development of motor milestones and increase muscle tone. Therapists who devote time to cooperative planning will find that one activity often provides therapy for the goals of each discipline. Moreover, the professionals who are not confined by the arbitrary boundaries of their respective disciplines can become more effective in serving the needs of the whole child (Edwards & Sparks, 1982; Harris, 1981).

Neurodevelopmental techniques have been applied in the treatment of dysfunctions of the central nervous system, such as cerebral palsy or trauma (Bobath, 1971; Trombley & Scott, 1977). The approach with Down syndrome applies the techniques to an immature nervous system instead of a damaged one. For example, the ability to sit up with adequate posture facilitates adequate breath support for speech. Therefore, techniques that strengthen the ability to sit without falling or slumping also further speech goals. Other goals are to increase muscle tone in the face, develop lip and jaw muscles for lip closure, and refine tongue movements for articulation. Techniques for these goals include a variety of early feeding activities of sucking, chewing, biting, touching the hard palate with the tongue, improving jaw strength, and swallowing without extending the tongue. Some examples of prelinguistic interdisciplinary therapy for Down syndrome are outlined below (Edwards, Sparks, Eidsvoog, Schmidt & Allen, 1983).

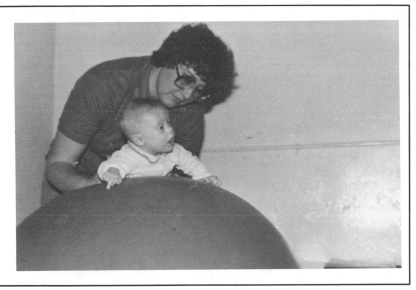

FIGURE 2-1
Three-month-old child with Down syndrome looks toward sound source from a therapy ball.

Goals for an infant at 3 to 4 months are: (a) increase muscle tone; (b) improve head control; (c) localize to noise for sound awareness. *Activity:* While lying on his stomach on the therapy ball, the child will lift his head to localize to a noisy toy. The speech clinician will present the noisy toy while the occupational therapist positions the child's weight on his arms, facilitating the child's head lifting.

Goals for prelinguistic behavior therapy at 0 to 12 months supported by research are establishing eye contact, turn taking, imitation, and expansion of utterances. Eye contact is encouraged by positioning the child face to face with the clinician for vocal play. Interruption of the child's vocal play with an imitation of his utterances will encourage turn-taking and imitation of the clinician's utterances.

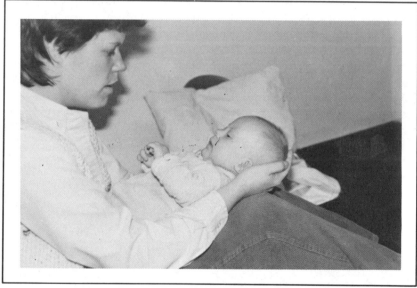

FIGURE 2-2
Vocal play with baby with Down syndrome. The clinician establishes eye contact and imitation.

Goals at 12 to 24 months are: (a) increase reaching; (b) increase trunk rotation; (c) increase attending behavior; (d) increase word production. *Activity:* The child will watch as the clinician blows bubbles to the child's left and then right side. The child will turn the upper portion of his body in order to pop the bubbles with his fingers. The clinician will wait for the child to say "more" before more bubbles are blown.

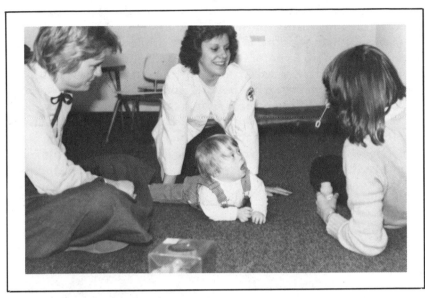

FIGURE 2-3
Two-year-old boy with Down syndrome must turn his body to pop bubbles and vocalize to initiate the activity.

The activity of eating a popsicle has several therapy goals: (a) The child vocalizes before each bite; (b) he increases muscle tone in his tongue and lips; (c) he is positioned for proper posture and balance.

Suggestions for therapy can be found in Hanson (1977), Schafer and Moersch (1981), and Dmitriev (1982). The following report of interdisciplinary therapy is an illustration of typical differences in motor and speech behavior of Down syndrome children.

Case Reports

Charley and Steve, two boys with Down syndrome, both nearly 2 years old, received interdisciplinary therapy from a speech-language pathologist and an occupational therapist for two 1-hour sessions per week. Although they were nearly identical in age, the boys were very different in behavior. Charley had better muscle tone and was very active. He spent the sessions in motion, usually walking around the room, climbing the steps, or climbing on the furniture. He mastered blowing bubbles in the water through a straw and through a wire loop to improve tone in the speech musculature. His oral expressive language was práctically nonexistent, but he used gestures well. Steve, on the other hand, spent the therapy sessions sitting on the floor unless coaxed and prodded to cruise (walk with support) around the furniture or to reach for objects. He was more hypotonic but more verbal than Charley. Steve learned to use five words consistently during the 4 months of therapy: mama, more, ball, bubble, and bye. The boys watched each other intently and often imitated one another. Charley seemed to spend all his energies to maintain his level of motor activity while Steve sat still and practiced his language.

A typical pattern in Down syndrome appears to be for language to emerge balanced by a temporary plateau in motor development and vice versa. Progress in either motor or speech behavior may be accompanied by an expected plateau in development of the other behavior.

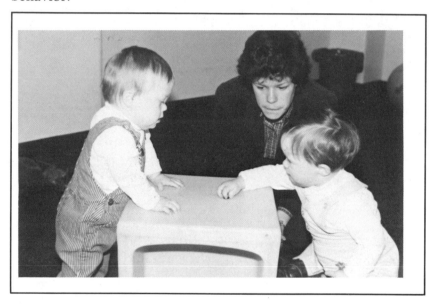

FIGURE 2-4
Two-year-old boys with Down syndrome imitate each other.

Phonological development

Recent researchers (Dodd, 1975; B.L. Smith & Stoel-Gammon, 1983; Stoel-Gammon, 1980) analyzed the speech of Down syndrome children for error types and phonological processes (substitution of one class of sounds for another, deletion of a class of sounds in a particular position in a word, and assimilation of one

sound by another). The studies agreed that the phonological processes and majority of errors of Down syndrome children were
similar to those reported for younger, normally developing
children. The Down syndrome children made more errors than
normal children did and their errors were less consistent. The
most commonly occurring errors were cluster reduction, gliding,
deletions of /h/ in all positions and nasals and liquids /l, r/ in final
position. Classes of sounds that had the highest number of correct
productions were stops /p, b, t, d, k, g/ and nasals /m, n, ng/ with the
exception of final position. B.L. Smith and Stoel-Gammon (1983)
studied the development of the use of plosives in the speech of five
Down syndrome children and found that they fell progressively
farther behind normal children during the first 4 years of
phonological development even though all the Down syndrome
children made improvements in their plosive use. This evidence
suggests that the phonological deficit, at least in plosive productions, is cumulative.

Articulation therapy

The above studies address two important issues for the clinician:
the errors of Down syndrome children have patterns, and the
error patterns are similar to those of normal children. It would
seem to follow that the same therapy techniques can be used that
are used with normal children. However, the clinician must
remember the physical differences in the visual and auditory
systems as well as the anatomical differences in the speech structures of Down syndrome children. Auditory discrimination skills
are weak, and material may be more easily learned visually. When
presenting new phonemes, clinicians may have more success if
those phonemes are associated with visual symbols rather than
relying on traditional auditory discrimination activities. Stop consonants and nasals are areas of strength and should be developed
fully for consistency and intelligibility.

Language development

Studies by several authors (Blanchard, 1964; Dodd, 1975;
Fisher, 1975) have found that virtually all Down syndrome
children have language deficits even though they may not have
defective articulation. Dodd further found that Down syndrome
children were better at pointing to an object when they heard it
named (visual modality) than were other retarded groups, but they
had more difficulty repeating words when there was a delay of 15

to 30 sec before the word was requested (auditory modality). Mein (1964) found that Down syndrome children have a higher proportion of nouns in their vocabularies than do normal children and showed strength in their abilities to express ideas through gestures and to understand pictures. They have great difficulty in comprehending negatives (Semmel & Dolley, 1971). The order of acquisition of morphemes by Down syndrome children was shown to correlate with R. Brown's (1973) developmental order of morpheme acquisition for normal children, although the age of acquisition was consistently later for Down syndrome children.

Language therapy

Perhaps the abundance of nouns in the vocabularies of Down syndrome children is due to the strength of their visual learning. Verbs and morphemes, in their developmental sequence, and articles and determiners should receive particular attention in therapy to counteract the typical "telegraphic speech" patterns in which these forms are omitted.

OTHER AUTOSOMAL CHROMOSOME SYNDROMES

Other syndromes with partial deletions or trisomies of autosomal chromosomes are too numerous for this discussion. Many, particularly trisomies of chromosomes 18, 13, and 8, have a limited chance for survival with death most often occurring within the 1st year (Nyhan, 1983). A few of those chromosomal anomalies that have good prognoses for survival have recently been studied for characteristic speech and language patterns.

Partial Trisomy 9p Syndrome

Owens and Beatty-Desana (1981) studied the speech and language of four subjects aged 4 years to 20 years who had a partial trisomy of chromosome 9 (two normal chromosomes plus an additional upper arm of chromosome 9). Characteristic features are mental retardation; short stature; delayed puberty; large, low-set ears; short hands with stubby fingers, simian palm creases, curved little fingers, and underdeveloped nails; and atypical facial features including antimongoloid eye slant, deep-set eyes, globular or beaked prominent nose, down-turned mouth, and high arched palate. These children with trisomy 9p exhibited receptive language consistent with overall retardation but with particularly poor expressive speech-language skills. Regardless of chronological age and receptive language age equivalents, the children used only consonant-vowel or vowel-consonant combinations to approximate words and did not combine words. It must be noted that a standardized test, the Sequenced Inventory of Communication Development (SICD) was given to only two of the four subjects. There was evidence of poor oral-motor coordination despite an essentially normal oral structure. All of the children tended to rely on gestures for communication. Three children received speech-language therapy for up to 2 years with no significant change in oral expression. Although this study had only four subjects, it is in basic agreement with an earlier study in which the authors concluded that the speech patterns of children with partial trisomy 9p syndrome were inconsistent with the degree of mental retardation (Zaremba, Zdienicka, Glogowska, Abramovicz, & Taracha, 1974). The reason for the characteristic receptive-expressive discrepancy is open to speculation encompassing lack of coordination of the oral musculature to auditory processing difficulties.

5p – , or Cri du Chat Syndrome

In this syndrome a birth cry, mewing and monotonic, about one octave higher than a healthy newborn's cry, is the diagnostic feature. The cat cry has been present in all of the cases found by karyotype to have partial deletion of the short arm of chromosome 5 (5p –).

Schinzel (1976) summarized the characteristics of the syndrome as low birth weight; growth retardation; mental retardation; round face with hypertelorism; epicanthic folds; antimongoloid positioning of the eyes; strabismus; receding chin; and short, tapering hands with small, incurving fingers. Some cases exhibit respiratory stridor (Niebuhr, 1971). Several authors described affected children as being "floppy" as infants and clumsy and awkward as they grew. Fussiness in infancy and rhythmic head-banging persisting into childhood were also mentioned in some cases (Dumars, Gaskill, & Kitzmiller, 1964; MacIntyre, Staples, La Polla, & Hempel, 1964; Schlegel, Neu, Carneiro Leao, Reiss, Nolan & Gardner, 1967). Schinzel (1976) described the gait as mostly unsteady and broad based but reported neurological signs as unremarkable.

Mental retardation is pronounced with cri du chat syndrome. Up to 1 % of the profoundly retarded (less than 20 IQ) are thought to have this syndrome (Bergsma, 1979). Breg and Steel (1970) studied 13 institutionalized patients aged 12 to 55 years. Of these, nearly all were unable to communicate. The catlike cry had disappeared and new features appeared: thin face, dental malocclusion, short metacarpals and metatarsals, scoliosis, small wings of the ilia, and prematurely gray hair. General health was good, but most had poor muscular development. Breg and Steel noted that there was considerable clinical variability in patients. They agreed with Moor (1968) that the mental retardation increases with age, but neither study cited data on IQ levels.

Ward, Engel, and Nance (1968) believe that the larynx becomes more normal as the child grows older. The long, curved, floppy epiglottis and the narrow diamond-shaped appearance of the glottis with an abnormally large air space in the posterior commissure area during phonation are responsible for a stridor and the catlike cry. During inspiration the elongated epiglottis flops down over the larynx, causing the stridor. During phonation and crying, the voice is weakened by air leakage because of the failure of the cords to approximate posteriorly, and the high-pitched cry is emitted from the approximated anterior portion of the cords.

Ward et al. (1968) reported four cases that show a typically severe pattern of expression of cri du chat syndrome. None of the children aged 1, 4, 8, and 12, had developed language. All four fell below the 10th percentile for their age in height and weight, and none could sit or walk unassisted.

Schlegel et al. (1967) reported an exceptional case of a 10-year-old girl with cri du chat syndrome with a full-scale Stanford Binet IQ of 58. She sat without aid at 3 years, and walked alone at 4 years, but was not yet toilet trained. Receptive language abilities were at about the level of a 3-year-old child. She did not respond to complex or two-step commands. Expressively she was echolalic. Her articulation was characterized by substitutions and omissions of sounds, but she did use actual words, not jargon. All nonverbal performance levels were severely retarded. Her voice was high-pitched and whining. A sonogram was prepared from her recorded speech and revealed "the vocalizations had little energy in the higher harmonics, had excessive breathiness at the conclusion of each vocalization, and were generally consistent with what is found with a hypotonic larynx" (p.5).

Case Report

Sparks and Hutchinson (1980) provide the following case report. Carolyn weighed 5 lb at birth. Her mother was 31 and her father was 33. Pregnancy was uncomplicated and full term with normal delivery. There were no congenital anomalies in the family history. She has one older sister who is normal. Cri du chat syn-

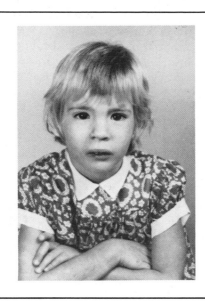

FIGURE 2-5
Four-year-old girl with cri du chat syndrome. Note hypertelorism, epicanthic folds, micronathia.

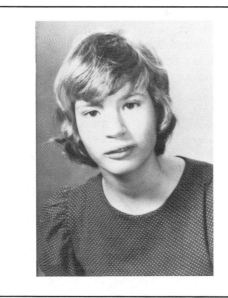

FIGURE 2-6
Same girl at age 13. Prosthetic bridge has replaced her incisors.

drome was suspected at birth due to a weak cry, which the physician said sounded like a mouse. Her palate was high and vaulted. Bottle feeding was impossible and nourishment was taken directly from a cup. A karyotype showed that Carolyn had a partial deletion of chromosome 5. Carolyn was also noted to have the facial appearance and microcephaly of cri du chat syndrome. On neurological examination, she tended to arch her back and was hyperflexic.

Carolyn's mother kept a detailed diary of her development. She was not fussy as a baby, but her small size and floppiness were a problem. It was hard to find toys small enough for her hands and chairs small enough for her to sit in. At 7 months she was still in birth-sized clothes. At 8 months she sat alone and attempted to say "ma-ma." A stridor was noted at night. She engaged in rhythmic head-banging and rocking. At 9 months she had a receptive vocabulary of 6 to 12 words. She crawled at 9 months, and at 17 months she began to pull herself to a standing position and to crawl up and down stairs. Her fine motor control appeared better than her gross motor control. The Cattell Infant Intelligence Scale was administered at 8 months and IQ range was estimated to be 50-65. The same test was repeated at 22 months with a resultant IQ of 52. She had pneumonia and meningitis at 22 months, and a plateau in development was noted. She walked at 26 months, before she could stand still.

Carolyn began speech therapy at the age of 31 months at the Charles Van Riper Language, Speech and Hearing Clinic, Department of Speech Pathology and Audiology at Western Michigan University.* She had an expressive vocabulary of approximately five words. At age 3, Carolyn entered a preschool special education program. She was using two-word phrases in school and at home. From ages 4 1/2 to 5 1/2 years, regressive behaviors appeared: silliness, sleep disturbances, and seemingly deliberate regression in toilet training. Speech and language development did not progress during that period. At age 4 years, 9 months her IQ (Stanford Binet) was 53. Her mental age on the Peabody Picture Vocabulary Test at age 5 years, 6 months was 2 years, 9 months. Regular pure-tone hearing test results were consistently within normal limits.

At age 7, Carolyn's IQ had regressed to 42 on the Stanford Binet, which is consistent with the progressive mental retardation found by Breg and Steel (1970) and Moor (1968). The Wechsler Intelligence Scale for Children (WISC) would have been the test of

---

* Hereafter referred to as WMU Speech, Language and Hearing Clinic.

choice, but the performance items were especially difficult for her due to her poor gross and fine motor control. Her voice was high pitched and weak with a fundamental frequency of 520 Hz compared to 273 Hz (Fairbanks, Herbert & Hammond, 1949) for normal females her age. Carolyn's use of speech phrases appeared to be limited more by her ability to sustain voicing than by her language ability. Her speech was telegraphic, but she had adequate functional language for her basic needs. She responded to three-part commands. Her articulation was characterized by substitutions and omissions. She tended to omit word endings and finished many phrases with a whisper (expiratory reserve).

At age 13, Carolyns's voice was still high pitched but it had lost much of the earlier breathiness. She used complete sentences. Her speech exhibited a strained rhythm pattern resembling that of cerebral palsy. The vowel sounds were prolonged, and the consonants were omitted or had soft contacts, particularly in the initial position. She was intelligible to her family but usually not to strangers. She was capable of her own care and some household duties. Speech therapy was part of her program in a class for the trainable mentally impaired.

In this child, who received excellent social and language stimulation from her family, early and consistent speech therapy, and special education, speech and language development surpassed that in all other reported cases (Schlegel et al., 1967; Ward et al., 1968) although physical and mental development were consistent with other cases. Her case may be unique but is reported here as evidence that speech and language therapy are warranted in cri du chat syndrome. Language patterns seem to be consistent with severe mental retardation, and language therapy should be focused on basic needs with limited goals. The unusual characteristic of cri du chat syndrome is the voice quality and very limited breath support. Attempts to alter the high pitch of the voice will likely be frustrating due to the unusual laryngeal structures. However, therapy to increase breath support should be a therapy goal. Speech production may be limited as much by the ability to maintain phonation as by limited language.

Partial Deletion of 15q, or Prader-Willi Syndrome

Prader-Willi syndrome consists of muscular hypotonia, obesity, short stature, small hands and feet, hypogonadism, and mental retardation (Ledbetter et al., 1981). Karyotypes of many patients with Prader-Willi syndrome have revealed a very small deletion in certain bands on chromosome 15, but its etiology may in fact be heterogeneous (Nyhan, 1983). Only the appearance of features of the syndrome permits definitive diagnosis if the deletion of chromosome 15 is not evident in the karyotype; thus, the diagnosis for a child may be in doubt for several years. Most often, Prader-Willi syndrome is diagnosed in late childhood, or even in adulthood, following referral for obesity. Obesity may be observed as early as 2 years of age, but it may not be extreme enough to warrant attention until the 3rd to 5th year. Hypotonia is striking from birth, and the mother may report weak fetal movements. The syndrome may cause respiratory or feeding problems, and tube feeding may be necessary in infancy.

Mental retardation is typical, (average IQ is 55) with some exceptions (Nyhan, 1983). Control over emotions appears to be deficient with extreme mood swings exhibited. No characteristic speech and language patterns typical of Prader-Willi syndrome have been described, but children or adults with this disorder may require therapy for delayed language consistent with the extent of retardation. Behavior is bizarre and centered around efforts to obtain food. Food must never be used as a reinforcement in Prader-Willi syndrome.

Summary

The severity of the physical and mental symptoms of the autosomal chromosome disorders of trisomy, nondisjunction, and translocation is a result of the large amount of genetic material involved. In contrast, in some individuals with Prader-Willi syndrome, the amount of deleted chromosomal material is comparatively small, and the symptoms are specific to a behavior disorder with either mild mental deficiency or normal intelligence. Even though there are general features dictated by the syndrome, individual differences exist in cognition, behavior, and rate of development. Clinicians must explore the anatomical and physical differences of these patients that affect the motoric aspects of speech production. The symptoms are stable, and gains made in therapy may be expected to be retained. Very early intervention programs with attention to development of the central nervous system offer promise for these children to attain their fullest potential.

SEX CHROMOSOME ANOMALIES

In the last 25 years, the process of chromosome banding has uncovered a variety of sex chromosomal anomalies associated with mental retardation and characteristic speech and language patterns. Sex chromosome abnormalities in boys may also be linked to an increased incidence of criminality (Nielsen, Sillesen, Sorensen, & Sorensen, 1979; Nyhan, 1983). Speech and language development have been studied extensively in children with sex chromosome abnormalities (Nielsen et al, 1979; A. Robinson, Lubs, Nielsen & Sorenson, 1979; Tennes, Puck, Orfanakis, & Robinson, 1977; Warkany, 1981). The information is summarized in Table 2-1. Of the children studied who had sex chromosome anomalies, there were some in whom no abnormality of growth, behavior or intelligence has been detected so far. It appears that the presence of an additional sex chromosome does not always disturb development, but rather may combine with genetic and environmental factors to produce susceptibility for a number of minor abnormalities in a threshold effect. The frequency of these children requiring speech therapy, especially those with 47,XXX (triple X) and 47,XXY, is high. The clinician should consider any child with a sex chromosome anomaly to be at risk for future language delay. Nielsen et al. (1979) stress the importance of early diagnosis for girls with triple X in order to advise parents concerning social stimulation and treatment of language delay and motor coordination. Triple X girls are also more at risk for difficulties with reading, spelling, and learning processes in general. Girls with XO (Turner syndrome) are the least likely to require speech and language therapy of those with sex chromose anomalies. Early diagnosis for boys with XXY and XYY is also important, not only because of a high incidence of learning problems, but because of an increased risk of behavioral and psychiatric problems as well (Nyhan, 1983). The behavior problems may not be evident until the boy enters school.

CHROMOSOMAL SYNDROME	FEATURES	SPEECH AND LANGUAGE	REFERENCES
47, XXX Girls	Usually normal appearance at birth; minor anomalies, such as epicanthic folds; passive; scanty facial expression; gives up easily; delayed gross and fine motor coordination; difficulties with peer group; delayed emotional maturity; withdrawn; slight increase in psychiatric problems	Delays in speech onset, combination of words, and expressive language; low scores on tests of verbal IQ; delay in mental & physical development until 4 to 8 years of age; problems with auditory discrimination; verbal expression and visual closure on Illinois Test of Psycholinguistic Abilities	Nielsen, et al., 1979 Robinson, et al., 1979
47,XXY Boys Klinefelter	One or more major congenital anomalies in 18% including cleft palate and nerve deafness; normal intellectual development apart from language; quiet; easy babies; scanty facial expression; withdrawn; distractible; delayed emotional maturity; minor psychiatric and school problems; gross motor delay but not fine motor	6-month delay in first words; delayed age for combining words; problems with expressive language and articulation; receptive language unaffected; strength in visual association; problem in auditory discrimination	Tennes, et al., 1977 Robinson, et al., 1979
47,XYY Boys	No phenotype but taller than average as adults; sometimes minor anomalies including abnormal ears, epicanthic folds, micrognathia; very active; needs demanding activity; aggressive; significantly increased number in penal & mental institutions	Slight decrease in verbal intelligence; normal to dull mentality	Robinson, et al., 1979 Tennes, et al., 1977
45 XO Turner Syndrome	Tendency to delay in emotional maturity; short stature; webbed neck; lack of sexual development	Perceptual hearing impairment; difficulty with auditory discrimination; mental retardation (10%); lower performance IQ than verbal IQ and full-scale IQ	Nielsen, et al., 1979 Warkany, 1981

TABLE 2-1.
Sex chromosome abnormalities.

Fragile X Syndrome

A rather subtle and, until very recently, easily missed abnormality of the X chromosome appears to be a relatively common cause of mental retardation. From one third to one half of all X-linked mental retardation is associated with the so-called fragile X chromosome, although there are isolated reports that the fragile X has been found in males who are not retarded. Next to trisomy 21, it is the most common of the causes of mental retardation that can be specifically diagnosed (Gerald, 1980; McKusick, 1978; Nyhan, 1983).

The discovery of fragile X began with the observation (Penrose, 1938) that there were 30 to 50% more males than females in institutions for the mentally retarded. This observation was repeatedly confirmed, leading to speculation that one or more undiagnosed forms of X-linked mental retardation might explain the anomalous sex ratio. Then Lubs (1969) described a family in which many members possessed an X chromosome with an unusually fragile, thin stalk, which was often broken. All male members of this family who possessed the fragile X chromosome were found to be mentally retarded. The genetic term for this fragile site is described as fra (X) (q27 or 28). The usual IQ range of these individuals is 20 to 70 (Turner, Daniel, & Frost, 1980).

Males with fragile X syndrome usually possess a few subtle phenotypic features, the most overt being enlargement of the testes after puberty to several times normal size (macro-orchidism). Although in other ways the males appear physically normal, careful examination during childhood may reveal minor variations: slightly increased head circumference; prominent forehead and jaw; long face; and enlarged ears (Turner, Brookwell, Daniel, Selikowitz & Zilibowitz, 1980).

There has been occasional mention of females heterozygous for the fragile X chromosome who were subnormal in intellectual development. Turner, Brookwell, Daniel, Selikowitz, and Zilibowitz (1980) concluded that expression of the X-linked mutation in female carriers contributes to mild mental retardation of girls. The female carrier has a 50% risk of having a son with moderate mental retardation.

Speech and language in fragile X syndrome

Howard-Peebles, Stoddard, and Mims (1979) studied adult members of four families with fragile X syndrome whose IQs ranged from 59 to 76. A generalized language disability was found, which tended to concentrate in the areas of auditory reception, auditory sequential memory, visual closure, and grammatic closure on the ITPA. Strengths were in nonverbal areas, such as manual expression and visual closure. None of the subjects had normal articulation. The most frequently occurring error was sound substitution, usually in the initial position, followed by omission, usually in the medial or final positions in words. Articulation errors involved the same sounds which are late in normal development and are misarticulated most frequently in the general population. None of the subjects had any anatomical abnormality of the speech mechanism, but some had difficulty with tongue control. The authors concluded that the misarticulations could be the result of delayed development and do not demonstrate a distinctive pattern.

Fragile X chromosome and autism

An isolated study by Brown et al. (1982) involved four males with previously established clinical diagnoses of autism. All four cases met the diagnostic criteria for autism: impaired social relationships, delayed and deviant language development, sterotyped or ritualistic behavior, and onset before the age of 30 months (Schopler & Dalldorf, 1980). All four subjects had fragile X syndrome leading the authors to speculate that the fragile X chromosome may show a significant frequency of association with autism. This study is interesting in light of the fairly recent discovery of fragile X but does not constitute sufficient evidence to link the two disorders without considerably more investigation.

Summary

Children and adults with known sex chromosome anomalies have been rare in the typical clinical case load. Recent evidence points to a higher incidence of sex chromosome disorders in the general population than was previously thought and, thus, may constitute a greater proportion of those who receive speech and language therapy, albeit undiagnosed, than clinicians have suspected. Furthermore, boys with fragile X chromosome may account for a surprising number of cases who exhibit moderate mental retardation. Individuals who have sex chromosome trisomies have characteristic speech and language patterns apart from mental retardation that may become apparent from a careful speech and language diagnostic evaluation. The importance of early diagnosis of the genetic abnormality by karyotype is evident for social and educational intervention. In fragile X, the speech and language patterns are consistent with general delayed development. An intriguing area for research is a suspected link between fragile X and autism.

REFERENCES

Ardran, G.M., Harker, P., & Kemp, P.T. Tongue size in Down syndrome. *Journal of Mental Deficiency Research*, 1972, 16, 160-166.

Bergsma, D. (Ed.), *Birth defects compendium* (2nd ed.). New York: Liss, 1979.

Blanchard, I. Speech patterns and etiology in mental retardation. *American Journal of Mental Deficiency*, 1964, 68, 612-617.

Bobath, B. *Abnormal postural reflex activity caused by brain lesions* (2nd ed.). London: William Heinemann Medical Books, 1971.

Breg, W.R., & Steel, M.W. The cri du chat syndrome in adolescents and adults: Clinical findings of thirteen older patients with partial deletion of the short arm of chromosome no. 5 (5p –). *Journal of Pediatrics*, 1970, 77, 782-791.

Brown, R. *First language, the early stages.* Cambridge, MA: Harvard University Press, 1973.

Brown, W.T., Friedman, E., Jenkins, E.C., Brooks, J., Wisniewski, K., Raguthu, S., & French, J.H. Association of fragile X syndrome with autism. *Lancet*, 1982, 1, 100.

Burch, P.R.J., & Milunsky, A. Early-onset diabetes mellitus in the general and Down syndrome populations. Genetics, etiology, and pathogenesis. *Lancet*, 1969, 1, 554-558.

Coleman, M., Schwartz, R.H., & Schwartz, D.M. Otologic manifestations in Down syndrome. *Down Syndrome Papers and Abstracts for the Professional*, 1979, 2(1), 1-2.

Dodd, B. Recognition and reproduction of words by Down syndrome and non-Down syndrome children. *American Journal of Mental Deficiency*, 1975, 80, 306-311.

Dmitriev, V. *Time to begin.* Milton, WA: Caring, 1982.

Dumars, K.W., Gaskill, C., & Kitzmiller, N. Le cri du chat (crying cat) syndrome. *American Journal of Diseases of Children*, 1964, 108, 533-542.

Edwards, S., & Sparks, S. *Intervention strategies for one Down syndrome twin: An interdisciplinary model.* Presentation of videotape, North Central Convention of the American Speech and Hearing Association, Milwaukee, WI, August, 1982.

Edwards, S., Sparks, S., Eidsvoog, M., Schmidt, L., & Allen, J. *Interdisciplinary techniques for Down syndrome.* Unpublished research, 1983.

Fairbanks, G., Herbert, E.L., & Hammond, J.H. An acoustical study of vocal pitch of seven and eight-year-old girls. *Child Development*, 1949, 20, 71-78.

Fisher, K. Mental development in mosaic Down syndrome as compared with trisomy 21. In R. Koch & F.F. de la Cruz (Eds.), *Down syndrome (mongolism) research prevention and management.* New York: Brunner/Mazel, 1975.

Gerald, P. X-linked mental retardation and an X-chromosome marker. *New England Journal of Medicine*, 1980, *303*(12), 696-697.

Hanson, M. *Teaching your Down syndrome infant*. Baltimore: University Park Press, 1977.

Harris, S. Effects of neurodevelopmental therapy on motor performance of infants with Down's syndrome. *Developmental Medicine and Child Neurology*, 1981, *23*, 477-483.

Heston, L.L. Alzheimer's disease, trisomy 21 and myeloproliferative disorders: Associations suggesting a genetic diathesis. *Science*, 1977, *196*, 322-323.

Howard-Peebles, P., Stoddard, G., & Mims, M. Familial X-linked mental retardation, verbal disability and marker X chromosomes. *American Journal of Genetics*, 1979, *31*, 214-222.

Jones, O.H.M. Prelinguistic communication skills in Down syndrome and normal infants. In T.M. Field (Ed.) *High risk infants and children: Adult and peer interactions* (pp. 205-225), New York: Academic Press, 1980.

Kirk, S., & Gallagher, J. *Educating exceptional children*. Boston: Houghton Mifflin, 1979.

Ledbetter, B.S., Ricardi, V.M., Airhart, S.D., Strobel, R.J., Keenan, B.S., & Crawford, J.D. Deletions of chromosome 15 as a cause of Prader-Willi syndrome. *New England Journal of Medicine*, 1981, *34*(6), 325-329.

Lenneberg, E.H., Nichols, I.A., & Rosenberger, E.F. Primitive stages of language development in mongolism. In D.M. Rioch and E.A. Weinstein (Eds.), *Proceedings of the Association for Research in Nervous and Mental Disease* (pp.119-137). Baltimore: Williams and Wilkins, 1964.

Lubs, H.A. A marker X chromosome. *American Journal of Human Genetics*, 1969, *21*, 231-244.

MacIntyre, M.N., Staples, W.I., La Polla, J., & Hempel, J.M. The "cat cry" syndrome. *American Journal of Diseases of Children*, 1964, *108*, 538-542.

McKusick, V.A. *Mendelian inheritance in man* (5th ed.). Baltimore: Johns Hopkins University Press, 1978.

Mein, R. A study of oral vocabularies of severely subnormal patients. *American Journal of Mental Deficiency*, 1964, *5*, 52-59.

Moor, L. L'asseration mentale dans le syndrome du cri du chat. *Revue de Neuropsychiatrie Infantile et d' hygiene mentale de l' Enfance*, 1968, *16*, 257.

Niebuhr, E. The cat cry syndrome (5p−) in adolescents and adults. *Journal of Mental Deficiency Research*, 1971, *4*, 277-291.

Nielsen, J., Sillesen, I., Sorensen, A.M., & Sorensen, K. Follow-up until ages 4 to 8 of 25 unselected children with sex chromosome abnormalities compared with sibs and controls. *Birth Defects*, 1979, *15*(1) 15-73.

Nyhan, W.L. Cytogenetic diseases. *Clinical Symposia*, Ciba, West Caldwell, NJ, 1983, *35*(1).

Owens, A., & Beatty-Desana, J. Communication functioning in trisomy 9p. *Journal of Communication Disorders*, 1981, *14*, 113-122.

Penrose, L.S. *A clinical and genetic study of 1,280 cases of mental defect* (Special report series no. 299). London: Medical Research Council, 1938.

Robinson, A., Lubs, H.A., Nielsen, J., & Sorensen, K. Summary of clinical findings: Profiles of children with 47,XXX, 47,XXY, and 47,XYY karyotypes. *Birth Defects*, 1979, 15(1) 261-266.

Robinson, N.M., & Robinson, H.B. *The mentally retarded child.* New York: McGraw-Hill, 1976.

Rowley, J.D. Down syndrome and acute leukemia: Increased risk may be due to trisomy 21. *Lancet*, 1981, 2(8254), 1020-22.

Schafer, D.S., & Moersch, M.S. (Ed.), *Developmental programming for infants and young children.* Ann Arbor: University of Michigan Press, 1981.

Schinzel, A. Autosomal chromosome aberrations. A review of the clinical syndromes caused by structural chromosome aberrations, mosaic trisomies 8 and 9, and triploidy. *Ergeb Inn Med Kinderheilkd*, 1976, 38, 37-94.

Schlegel, R.J., Neu, R.L., Carneiro Leao L., Reiss, J.A., Nolan, T.B., & Gardner, L.I. Cri du chat syndrome in a 10 year old girl with deletion of the short arms of chromosome number 5. *Helvetica Paediatrica Acta*, 1967, 22, 2-12.

Schopler, E., & Dalldorf, J. Autism: Definition, diagnosis and management. *Hospital Practice*, 1980, 15, 64-73.

Scoggin, C.H., & Patterson, D. Down syndrome as a model disease. *Archives of Internal Medicine*, 1982, 142, 462-464.

Semmel, M., & Dolley, D. Comprehension and imitation of sentences by Down syndrome children as a function of transformational complexity. *American Journal of Mental Deficiency*, 1971, 75, 739-745.

Smith, B.L. *Phonological development in Down syndrome children.* Paper presented at the Symposium of the American Psychological Society, San Francisco, 1977.

Smith, B.L., & Oller, D.K. A comparative study of pre-meaningful vocalizations produced by normally developing and Down syndrome infants. *Journal of Speech and Hearing Disorders*, 1981, 46, 46-51.

Smith, B.L., & Stoel-Gammon, C. A longitudinal study of the development of stop consonant production in normal and Down's syndrome children. *Journal of Speech and Hearing Disorders*, 1983, 48(2), 114-118.

Smith, D.W. *Recognizable patterns of human malformation. Genetic, embryologic and clinical aspects* (3rd ed.), Philadelphia: Saunders, 1982.

Smith, D.W., & Wilson, A.A. *The child with Down syndrome.* Philadelphia: Saunders, 1973.

Sparks, S., & Hutchinson, B. Cri du chat: Report of a case. *Journal of Communication Disorders*, 1980, 13, 9-13.

Stoel-Gammon, C. Phonological analysis of four Down syndrome children. *Applied Psycholinguistics*, 1980, 1, 31-48.

Stoel-Gammon, C. Speech development of infants and children with Down syndrome. In J. Darby, Jr. (Ed.), *Speech evaluation in medicine* (pp. 341-360). New York: Grune & Stratton, 1981.

Tennes, K., Puck, M., Orfanakis, D., & Robinson, A. The early childhood development of 17 boys with sex chromosome anomalies: A prospective study. *Pediatrics*, 1977, 59(4), 574-583.

Thompson, J.S., & Thompson, M.W. *Genetics in medicine.* Philadelphia: Saunders, 1980.

Trombley, C., & Scott, D. *Occupational therapy for physical dysfunction.* Baltimore: Williams and Wilkins, 1977.

Turner, G., Brookwell, R., Daniel, A., Selikowitz, M., & Zilibowitz, M. Heterozygous expression of X-linked mental retardation and X-chromosome marker fra(X) (q 27). *New England Journal of Medicine*, 1980, 303(12), 662-664.

Turner, G., Daniel, A., & Frost, M. X-linked mental retardation, macro-orchidism and the Xq27 fragile site. *Journal of Pediatrics*, 1980, 96, 837-841.

Ward, P., Engel, E., & Nance, W. The larynx in cri du chat (cat cry) syndrome. *Laryngoscope*, 1968, 78, 1716-1733.

Warkany, J., Chromosomal syndromes. In J. Warkany, R.J. Lemire, & M.M. Cohen, Jr. (Eds.), *Mental retardation and congenital malformations of the central nervous system.* Chicago: Year Book Medical, 1981.

Zaremba, J., Zdienicka, E., Glogowska, I., Abramovicz, T., & Taracha, B. Four cases of 9p trisomy resulting from a balanced familial translocation (9;15)(q13;q11). Clinical picture and cytogenetic findings. *Journal of Mental Deficiency Research*, 1974, 18, 153-190.

3

Single-Gene Disorders

Single-gene disorders are caused by altered forms of genes (mutations). A mutation results in a problem for the proband in two ways: the altered gene must be present on both chromosomes of a pair in recessive disorders or present on only one chromosome of a pair and matched with a normal gene on the partner chromosome in autosomal dominant and sex-linked disorders. In either case, the cause of the defect is a single major error in the genetic blueprint. Single-gene disorders usually exhibit obvious and characteristic pedigree patterns of transmission (see Chapter 1) (Thompson & Thompson, 1980). In this chapter, some representative single-gene disorders that involve primary growth deficiency and characteristic speech and language patterns are presented in some detail, along with case histories.

RECESSIVE GENE DISORDERS

Over the past 80 years, 521 autosomal recessive disorders have been described, and there are 596 more disorders in which the possibility of recessive transmission exists (McKusick, 1978). Recessive disorders tend to have less variation in expression than do autosomal dominant disorders, possibly because both genes of a pair are mutant, and there is no normal partner gene to carry on the function of the gene (Smith, 1982). Of the recessive disorders, 160 different kinds are now known to be caused by a biochemical abnormality in the gene responsible for directing the production of an *enzyme*. The gene functions incorrectly or not at all, leading to what are known as *inborn errors of metabolism* (Apgar & Beck, 1972; Summer & Shoaf, 1982).

Enzymes are involved in the complex chemical reactions by which the food an individual eats is transformed into energy, body tissue, and waste products (metabolism). Some essential substances needed by the body must be produced out of chemicals in food, and every reaction takes place by many interrelated steps. When an enzyme is missing or is abnormally made because of a defective gene, the orderly steps in the process of metabolism are disrupted. The absence of an enzyme may prevent a normal reaction from taking place or may bring about a reaction that ordinarily does not take place, that is, some substance will not be formed that should be formed, or it will be formed in excessive amounts, which may, in turn, affect the workings of other enzymes or the function of body organs. Any interference with enzyme action, at almost any point, will set off a chain reaction (Azimov, 1962). For example, if the specific enzyme needed to turn Compound A into Substance B is missing, Compound A may accumulate in the body to such a high level that it causes cell damage directly, or it may be made into abnormal products by other enzymes that are not normally active in breaking down this material. The critical factors in severity of a disorder are the degree to which the function of the organs where the material is stored is disturbed and the toxicity of the product that is produced. Inborn errors of metabolism are diverse, representing a wide variety of enzyme defects. In the phenotype, the disorders range in severity from relatively harmless to those causing mental retardation, as in phenylketonuria (PKU) and Sjogren-Larsson syndrome, or death, as in Hunter syndrome.

Sjogren-Larsson Syndrome and Histidinemia

In 1963, Witkop and Henry described speech and language patterns in two similar autosomal recessive, biochemical diseases, Sjogren-Larsson syndrome and histidinemia. The biochemical manifestation was aminoaciduria in which there was urinary excretion of large amounts of histidine plus arginine in the former disorder, and histidine in the latter.

In Sjogren-Larsson syndrome, the clinical manifestations similar to PKU are: mental retardation, ichthyosis (fish-scale skin), and spasticity in the extremities. The children described by these authors appeared to be normal at birth, except for the ichthyosis. At 4 to 8 months of age the symptoms appeared and were progressive. The speech pattern was distinctive and could not be accounted for by the retardation. "Some did not speak. Others showed hesitancy, stuttering, inarticulation, monotonous speech, substituting single words for whole sentences, mispronunciation of vowels, and the inability to put words into sentences. . . .Many patients kept their mouths open which was accompanied by drooling" (p.110). The severely affected children never sat or walked and retained strong sucking and rooting reflexes. The moderately affected children walked with a stumbling gait. They could understand and obey simple commands and communicated primarily with signs. Those who used single words had special difficulty in pronouncing /t/ and /s/ sounds and did not form sentences.

In histidinemia, mental retardation is milder than in Sjogren-Larsson syndrome. In these children consistent articulation problems appeared, which were accompanied by a deviation of the tongue tip to the right and orbicularis oris. There was an inability of the tongue to perform movements independent of the mandible. The second consistent problem was language errors of syntax and noun usage. They exhibited problems of memory and recall for verbal auditory symbols, suggesting central nervous system scrambling. The authors suggested an association of the genetic biochemical defect with a disorder of speech, language, and other oral functions.

This well done study is noteworthy for several reasons: It was a pioneer effort (1963) from the collaboration of a speech pathologist and a dentist at the National Institutes of Health, and it was the first to suggest that specific inborn errors of metabolism are related to specific speech behaviors. This study has withstood the test of time, and the presence of the speech patterns described is used by medical geneticists to diagnose these disorders.

X-LINKED RECESSIVE DISORDERS

There are 107 definite and 98 suspected disorders that are X-linked in which the abnormality is manifested only in the sons of carrier mothers (McKusick, 1978). A trait inherited as an X-linked recessive is expressed by all males who carry the gene. An X-linked trait may be transmitted through a series of carrier women before it appears in an affected male (Thompson & Thompson, 1980). The two disorders described here are called *genetic lethal* in that the nature of the disorder prevents its transmission by affected males, but it is spread by carrier females who themselves rarely show any manifestation of the disease.

Duchenne Muscular Dystrophy

No biochemical defect has been uncovered in this X-linked degenerative disease of muscle, which affects only males. There are recent suggestions that the disease may be due, in part, to neural or neuronal defects (Bergsma, 1979). It is marked by weakness of the involved muscles, first of the pelvic girdle, followed by the shoulder girdle and hypertrophy of the calf muscles. It is usually apparent by the time the child begins to walk and progresses so that he is confined to a wheelchair by about the age of 10 and is unlikely to survive his teens (Thompson & Thompson, 1980).

Karagan and Zellweger (1978) studied the early verbal and performance IQ (WISC) of 53 mildly disabled boys with Duchenne muscular dystrophy and found the full-scale IQ score was significantly below normal in all the subjects. Another important finding was a verbal-performance discrepancy with the mean verbal IQ (80.66) significantly lower than the mean performance IQ (88.06). These results agree with Marsh and Munsat (1974) that early verbal disability is a characteristic of Duchenne muscular dystrophy. The depressed scores could not be attributed to age or degree of physical disability. The authors suggest that the behavior may be related to the direct physical influence of the disease upon central nervous system functioning. The verbal disability is present at an early age when most young boys with Duchenne muscular dystrophy are only minimally restricted and are thus able to explore their environment. The implication for the clinician who works with a patient with this disorder is to expect a degree of very early verbal impairment more severe than the degree of physical impairment would indicate. Very limited language goals with the flexibility to change them as the disease progresses is imperative.

Hunter Syndrome (Mucopolysaccharidosis, or MPS)

Hunter syndrome is an X-linked recessive disorder in the group called lysosomal storage diseases, in which specific enzymes do not function to break down complex carbohydrates called mucopolysaccharides. As a consequence, mucopolysaccharides accumulate, and cells throughout the body where they are stored become distended and disrupted leading to gross functional disturbances (MPS Society; Young & Harper, 1981). The major physical characteristics are short stature with large head, stiff joints, involvement of the heart and other organs, atypical face, and coarse hair (Smith, 1982). The symptoms are progressive. These children have been described as gargoyles because of their alleged resemblance to the grotesque effigies on cathedrals in France. Other forms of MPS, all autosomal recessive but not X-linked, are Hurler, Scheie, Sanfilippo, Maroteaux, Sly, and Di Ferrante syndromes (Thompson & Thompson, 1980). They are all very similar in phenotype, although Hunter syndrome is usually milder. A disorder of MPS occurs in approximately 125 infants annually in the United States (Nadler, 1975).

There are two forms of Hunter syndrome (McKusick, 1978). In the mild form, the physical symptoms are present with normal or near normal intellect, and survival beyond 20 years is usual. In the severe form, the physical changes are accompanied by gross neurodegeneration with global retardation and regression. Survival beyond 15 years is rare. Clinicians should note that serious behavior problems are common. Young and Harper (1981) suggested that the various patterns of behavior are related to the cerebral damage from storage of mucopolysaccharides. They classified severe Hunter syndrome behavior into four categories:

1. Overactivity. Child is tireless and exhausting to others and has interrupted sleep patterns.

2. Obstinacy. Child is stubborn and has temper tantrums. If denied or thwarted, child will throw anything at hand.

3. Aggression. Child is antisocial, violent, and destructive. These problems are exacerbated by the rapid growth in the early years.

4. Exuberance. This behavior is less frequent than the other behaviors. Child is loveable and affectionate, playful, and eager to help. Disturbances result from over-enthusiasm rather than willful design.

No particular drug to modify behavior has been especially effective. Residential care is often the only alternative for affected individuals who have the severe behavioral disorders and physical problems that require total care. Behavioral disturbances are rare in the mild form, and custodial care is usually not warranted.

Children with the MPS disorders frequently have impaired hearing. Incidence of hearing loss is hard to estimate because of the difficulty in testing due to mental retardation. Many children have chronic serous otitis media and ossicular malformations, but a coexisting progressive sensorineural hearing loss is often not recognized (Hayes, Babin, & Platz, 1980). Audiometric examination should be routine and thorough. No information about specific speech and language patterns in Hunter syndrome is available, but it is reasonable that speech and language development would be influenced by the age of onset of the disorder and the degree of consequent mental retardation.

The Role of the Clinician in Progressive Lethal Disorders

The difference between the recessive diseases of Hunter syndrome and Duchenne muscular dystrophy and the chromosomal disorders discussed in Chapter 2 is the progression of the debilitating symptoms. Regression, not progress, is the expected

course. Such a prognosis poses some unique problems for the clinician for whom improvement is the expected course of therapy.

A common reaction of health-care professionals faced with the
frustration of patient decline is to withdraw; if nothing more can
be done, the clinician need not try. Withdrawal, which may appear to be an uncaring attitude, can also be found in many parents
of dying children. It is not lack of caring, but an inability and un-
willingness to witness the decline of the child. The family of such a
child needs a clinician who is realistic, who will be supportive,
who will discuss the current state of the child without denial of the
obvious conditions, and who will set realistic goals for therapy. If
the child cannot attain the objectives, they must be changed to fit
his changing abilities. Although it may seem too obvious to mention, clinicians in this unfamiliar situation who maintain
unrealistic pressure for improvement may bring about needless
frustration for the child, the parents, and themselves. The following case report illustrates typical clinician denial.

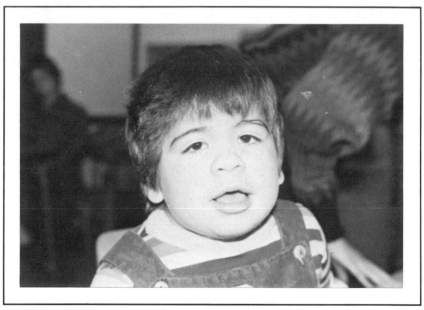

FIGURE 3-1.
Three-year-old boy with Hunter syndrome. Note large head and coarse
features.

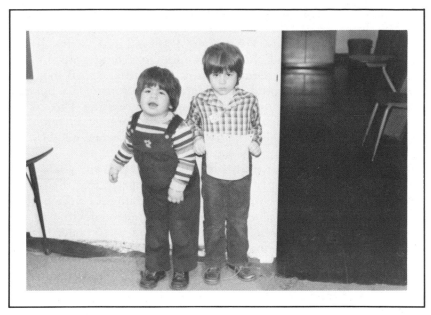

FIGURE 3-2.
Three-year-old boy with Hunter syndrome with normal 5-year-old brother.
Note body proportions.

Case Report

Mark was diagnosed at age 2 as having Hunter syndrome and began therapy at the WMU Speech, Language and Hearing Clinic a few months later. He weighed 58 lb at age 3 (the average weight for an 8 year old) and was as tall as his 5 year old normal brother. Mark's behavior fell into the exuberant classification (Young & Harper, 1981). Although he was active and had a short attention span, he was also affectionate and personable. His physical symptoms of poor motor coordination were complicated by Erb palsy (perinatal injury) that left his left side weak. His large size and clumsiness often resulted in materials being swept from the table or puzzles spilled onto the floor. In addition to speech therapy in the clinic, Mark went to a special education class each morning where he received structured language and speech therapy. Although Mark's receptive language seemed fairly good, his attention span was too short for formal testing. His expressive language consisted of one word utterances (holophrases) and gestures. For example, when he heard a train whistle, Mark pointed to the window, shook his head up and down and said, "Dad," which meant that his father had taken him to see a train. Mark particularly enjoyed imaginative play. He prepared, served and ate imaginary food and used his holophrases to talk to friends on the toy telephone. A hearing screening was conducted at 25 dB in sound field, because Mark would not tolerate earphones. His hearing appeared to be within normal limits on the screening. Due to the expected progressive hearing disorder in Hunter syndrome, his hearing will be tested often. Hearing aids are recommended by the audiologist at the first sign of hearing loss.

It became evident that traditional language therapy goals were proving to be frustrating and were not appropriate for this child. The level of his current communication skills might be the best he could achieve, and those skills were expected to decline in the course of his genetic disease. The main goal was to make Mark's communication skills enhance his quality of life and maintain those skills as long as possible. A meeting was held with his parents, school clinician and university clinician to decide on an alternative communication system to be used when even his holophrases would no longer be possible. Signing was eliminated because of his poor motor skills. Blissymbolics were introduced, but he was resistent and uncooperative when they were presented. Instead, a picture board was devised that contained pictures of Mark's family and basic things in his life. Two things were important in the choice of pictures for the board: the pictures needed to be identical for school, home, and clinic, so three identical boards were made; and pictures for the expression of feelings were included (love, happy, sad). The picture board was a required part of each therapy session even though it was apparent that as long as Mark could use speech and gestures, he would resist learning an alternate system.

In Mark's case the roles of the professional, who educates, and the parents, who must be educated, were reversed. The clinicians who worked with Mark were more supported by his mother than able to support her. Mark's mother was clear and pragmatic about communication goals for her child. She explained the expected course of Hunter syndrome to the clinicians: the decline in all areas of ability, loss of mobility and cognition, and death. The clinicians behaved as if that outcome was only a possibility or that, in this case, things would be different. It was his mother who suggested the alternative communication system and used the words "when he needs it," while the clinicians said "if he needs it."

At age 4 Mark is still making gains and maintaining previously learned skills. It could be speculated that Mark's lack of aberrant behaviors and good social interactions enable him to be a participating member of his family and school class for an unusually protracted period.

AUTOSOMAL DOMINANT DISORDERS

McKusick(1978) has cataloged 736 inherited defects that are definitely transmitted by autosomal dominant inheritance and a similar number that have been suspected of being inherited in this way (see Chapter 1 for inheritance pattern). However, spontaneous change can occur in which a dominant gene is not inherited but created new due to a change in a gene of an egg or a sperm. These "new mutations" produce affected offspring from normal parents. The proband then has the same risk of passing the dominant gene to his offspring as if it had been inherited (50%). Of special interest to clinicians is a group of autosomal dominant disorders that involve craniofacial anomalies with their speech and language problems.

Craniofacial Anomalies

The incidence of genetic craniofacial disorders other than cleft palate and cleft lip has been thought to be relatively low, but in recent years more of these patients have been reported, and new syndromes are being identified regularly.

Apert and Crouzon Syndromes

These disorders are very similar in that both have definitive abnormalities in the growth and shape of the skull due to craniostenosis (premature closure of one or more of the several sutures of the cranium) and facial malformations of hypertelorism, extreme protrusion of the eyes, and beaked nose. Apert syndrome is further characterized by anomalies of the fingers and toes. The cranial pressure from the growing brain must be relieved surgically to prevent mental retardation (Bergsma, 1979). The extent of the craniofacial abnormalities are not indicative of the extent of the mental defect, if any. Persons with severe external craniofacial malformations may be mentally normal, whereas persons with mild craniostenosis may be mentally defective because of associated brain anomalies. Bergstrom (1980) and Warkany (1981) note that children with Apert and Crouzon syndromes are prone to conductive hearing loss due to fixation of the ossicular chain and deformities of the external canal and of the eustachian tube. Children with Crouzon syndrome are typically less severely affected in all areas, including speech, and have a better prognosis for mental development than children with Apert syndrome.

Both disorders are dominant traits, but while few pedigrees are on record to show that Apert syndrome is transmitted from generation to generation, there are many observations of Crouzon syndrome that show such transmission. Most cases of Apert syndrome, therefore, are new mutations. The pedigrees of persons with Crouzon syndrome indicate that affected members are socially better accepted than are patients with Apert syndrome, and they can find work and mates with whom to pass on the condition to some of their children (Warkany, 1981).

There are similar characteristics of the speech structures in the two syndromes. The upper jaw is much smaller than the lower jaw, and there is severe malocclusion, high arched palate filled with soft tissue, and severely reduced size of the nasal airways. The voice quality is denasal, sometimes described as muffled (Peterson, 1973). In addition, some children have a cleft palate or a soft palate that is insufficient to close the nasal port for speech. Therefore, there is considerable reason to expect individuals with craniofacial anomalies to have dysarthrias due to deviations in the positions of the oral structures. But it is unclear what role the degree of deviation plays in the speech of these individuals. Many are able to compensate well for a high arched palate, misaligned teeth, and small or bowed jaw; others have much difficulty. Hearing loss, of which there is a high incidence in craniofacial anomalies, also interferes with the development of language. In addition, it seems possible that the psychosocial impact of the craniofacial anomaly may result in impaired social interaction and thus retard speech and language acquisition (Elfenbein, Waziri, & Morris, 1981).

Case Report

Robert weighed 8 1/2 lb at birth and was delivered with high forceps. His obviously malformed skull with a circumference of 38 cm (above the 95th percentile for newborn males), bulging temporal areas, thick coronal sutures, and hypertelorism led to a diagnosis of Crouzon syndrome. Surgeries to relieve the craniostenosis were performed beginning at 2 months, followed by four more operations between 5 and 7 months of age. The surgeon noted that Robert's brain expanded immediately during the first procedure. During one operation, cardiac arrest occurred due to a kink in the endotracheal tube. He was resuscitated immediately and recovered with no apparent damage.

Robert's parents were told by their physicians that their child probably would be retarded and probably would not walk or talk. They did not accept that prognosis and sought other medical and rehabilitative services. Robert was evaluated for speech therapy at age 3, and it was discovered that he had a severe conductive hearing loss (60 dB bilaterally) due to stenosis of the ear canals. His language was severely delayed at that time. He was fitted with hearing aids, which brought his thresholds to within normal limits. Robert made immediate progress in both expressive and receptive language after he received hearing aids.

At age 5, after five corrective surgeries, Robert was described as having an abnormally shaped head, a beaked nose, low-set ears and slight bulging of the eyes. He also had a Class III malocclusion (mesioclusion) with protruded mandible in relation to the maxilla and anterior open bite. His maxilla appeared to be tilted posteriorly-superiorly. Robert was able to chew with minimal retraction of the mandible. He had a high narrow palatal arch with slight lateral accumulations of soft tissue and a complete uvula. His nasal airways were considerably narrowed; his lips were habitually open, and respiration was audible. Vocal resonance varied from hyponasal to normal to hypernasal. Nasal emission of air on phonation was inconsistent. There were numerous sound substitutions, omissions, and distortions in his articulation. Receptive language was normal.

At age 6, Robert had another operation in which the bones of the middle third of his face were fractured and moved forward. Robert then had to accommodate the change in alignment of his articulators, having particular difficulty with contacts for plosives and articulatory precisions. Another surgery for stenosis of the ear canals is planned for a later time. He continued to require speech and language therapy and auditory training in the clinic and at school until he was in first grade.

There are three important implications for therapy in this child's case: the erroneous expectation of abnormal development, the undetected hearing loss during the critical period of language learning, and the identification of behaviors that were and those that were not amenable to change. Robert responded to intensive language therapy after he was fitted with hearing aids. Articulation therapy focused on teaching contacts that compensated for his misaligned structures. He achieved the goals that were within the realm of possibility given his deviant structures. There was no attempt to change those aspects of his speech that could not be changed, such as his denasal voice quality and some imprecision of articulation. The only special service that he continues to receive in school is monitoring by the consultant for the hearing impaired.

Treacher-Collins Syndrome

This relatively rare syndrome is autosomal dominant with almost 100% penetrance and 60% presumed new mutations (Smith, 1982). If a parent is affected, 50% of the offspring are at risk.

Individuals with Treacher-Collins syndrome exhibit a wide range of physical findings. Those that have particular bearing on speech and language include conductive and/or sensorineural hearing loss, very small underdeveloped jaws, high arched or cleft palate, and malocclusion. Treacher-Collins syndrome has the same phenotype as a sporadic syndrome called Goldenhar's syndrome. It is important that early diagnosis be made to differentiate the two syndromes. The child with Goldenhar's should be treated for preventable scoliosis, and the child with Treacher-Collins should have the possibility of hearing loss investigated immediately (Bergstrom, 1980). As the child with Treacher-Collins grows older, the curve of the jaw and open bite become worse. Speech and language characteristics include delayed language development consistent with hearing loss, articulatory defects, and hypernasality consistent with the craniofacial anomaly.

Johnston, Taussig, Koopman, Smith, and Bjelland (1981) report that children with Treacher-Collins syndrome frequently have sleep apnea. As the child sleeps, respiration grows progressively slower and may finally stop. The need for oxygen results in a gasping for breath and frequent awakening. The authors speculate that poor school performance, short attention span, and disruptive behaviors often seen in these children may be aggravated by sleep disturbances. Craniofacial surgery has been successful in improving self-image and speech and in eliminating the sleep apnea.

Treatment for Craniofacial Disorders

Treatment by a multidisciplinary team, such as in a center that traditionally treats oral cleft patients, is the logical place for these patients to be referred. The participation of a speech clinician on this team is critical, especially when a surgical correction is contemplated. Surgery to correct the face, known as facial osteotomy, is becoming more prevalent, particularly with Apert and Crouzon syndromes. Improvements in articulation after surgery have been documented by Witzel, Ross, and Munro (1980) and Glass, Knapp, and Bloomer (1977). Improved self-image as a result of improved appearance is an overriding reason for investigation of surgery. Careful audiologic evaluation is also necessary, as hearing loss often remains undetected.

Van der Woude Syndrome

The clinician who is part of an oral-cleft team should be aware of a genetic condition associated with lower lip pits. Van der Woude syndrome is an autosomal dominant condition with variable expression and incomplete penetrance (Smith, 1982). The expression most likely to bring a patient to the attention of the clinician is cleft lip or palate, but other symptoms are lip pits and submucous cleft. Glass, Stewart, and Miles (1979) reported a family in which some members had only lip pits, some had lip pits with a cleft of the lip and palate, and others had lip pits with a submucous cleft. One member of the family had been seen in an oral cleft clinic and the lip pits were noted. The family was not aware of the genetic nature of the disorder. Subsequent to investigation of the pedigree, other family members who had not been diagnosed previously, and who had associated speech disorders, received therapy. Family members at risk for transmission of the disorder received genetic counseling.

Huntington Disease

Huntington disease is an autosomal dominant neuro-degenerative disease in which the symptoms are choreiform movement, dementia, and psychiatric disturbance. The symptoms usually appear between the ages of 35 and 45, but a less common form afflicts children, sometimes as young as age 2 (National Institutes of Health, 1979). The course of the disease is more rapid in children, and they may die 8 to 10 years after onset. The older a person is when the symptoms begin, the milder the disease.

Huntington disease was once thought to be rare but is now recognized as one of the more common hereditary disorders. The incidence is about one in 25,000 (Thompson & Thompson, 1980), but approximately twice this number are at risk. New mutations are exceptionally rare; probably 95% of affected individuals receive the gene from an affected parent ("Genetic Counseling," 1982). It is difficult to obtain accurate incidence or prevalence rates for Huntington disease, because patients are often misdiagnosed as schizophrenic or as suffering from another neurological condition.

No laboratory test can positively identify the person with Huntington disease. Persons at risk must wait until symptoms appear to know if the gene is present, often after they have already completed their families. Early symptoms are almost imperceptible and may be mistaken for nervousness or irritability. Physical symptoms may first appear as tics, jerks, or spasms of the face and body. Speech may become slightly slurred or unsteady. As the disease progresses, mental and physical symptoms gradually increase. Small movements may become more exaggerated and extreme until all parts of the body are in constant uncontrollable motion. Swallowing becomes difficult, and choking is a hazard. Speech eventually slurs beyond comprehension. Death usually results from infection, heart failure, or choking.

Speech therapy may prolong the period of comprehensible speech. Patients may not be able to communicate their thoughts and needs as they lose the capacity to speak but usually retain their receptive abilities. When speech fails, alternative communication devices, such as electronic speech synthesizers, can be used to decrease the frustration and anger felt by the patients when they cannot make their needs known. Such devices must allow for the extreme motor problems of these patients.

The speech clinician may be part of a team of health professionals involved with the care of a Huntington disease patient. The role of the clinician in this disease, as in the other lethal disorders, is to be realistic and supportive. The patient and family should be cautioned that problems are almost inevitable in employment, marriage, and family and personal relationships (Shoulson & Fahn, 1979). Virtually all patients and families feel threatened by the fear of abandonment. It is helpful for the clinician to recognize these concerns and to acknowledge them.

SPORADIC DISORDERS

A trait is said to be *sporadic* when it occurs in a single individual in a family and has no known genetic basis (Thompson & Thompson, 1980). Although they are birth defects, these disorders should not be confused with new mutations of a dominant or recessive gene that can be transmitted. Three such disorders are reviewed here because of the speech and language disorders involved.

Möbius Syndrome

Möbius syndrome is a rare syndrome in which a sporadic basis is suspected (Smith, 1982). The characteristics include congenital, nonprogressive, usually bilateral facial paralysis of the sixth and seventh cranial nerves, and, frequently, involvement of other cranial nerves, such as the oculomotor, trigeminal and, especially, the hypoglossal. There may also be unilateral or bilateral loss of function of the abductors of the eye and anomalies of the extremities. Mental retardation is reported in 15% of the cases. (Bedrossian & Lachman, 1956; Gorlin & Pindborg, 1964; Smith, 1982). The most immediate problem arises in infancy, because the facial paralysis makes sucking nearly impossible. Deviant chewing and swallowing may continue to be a problem, depending on the involvement of other cranial nerves innervating the peripheral muscles of the tongue and jaw (Kahane, 1979). Individuals with Möbius syndrome have a masklike face. Their inability to smile or show facial expression is socially handicapping and gives the appearance of retardation. The paralysis makes it impossible to close the lips, and the mouth is characteristically held open. There is an expected absence of bilabial sounds /p, b, m/ from paralysis of orbicularis superioris. Other cranial nerves innervating the peripheral speech mechanism may also be involved in this disorder. If tongue atrophy restricts tongue mobility, the lingua-alveolar sounds /t, d, n/ may be produced as lingua-dentals (th). The lingua-velar sounds /k, g/ may be produced pharyngeally with the tongue resting on the floor of the mouth, and sibilants /s, sh/ and fricatives /f, v/ may be interdentalized (Kahane, 1979). Vowel productions may also be distorted by imprecise placement and restricted movements of the tongue during speech. Helmick (1980) reported increased difficulty with articulation when rapid speech was attempted. Helmick also reported a case in which resonance was markedly hypernasal as a result of paresis in the velopharyngeal region. Impaired innervation of the palate may render the tensor veli palatini an ineffective dilator of the eustachian tube, which may, in turn, lead to otitis media.

Therapy for the dysarthria caused from facial paralysis calls for compensatory articulatory movements. For the bilabial sounds, labiodental productions (contact of the lower lip with the incisors) may be substituted to produce a perceptually correct phoneme, that is, /m, p, b/ can be produced with the articulators in the position for /f/. Slow rate and overarticulation will help to increase intelligibility. To compensate for the lack of communicative facial expression, the child may be taught to vary the prosody of his speech.

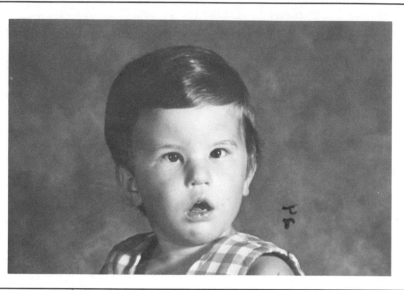

FIGURE 3-3.
Two-year-old boy with Möbius syndrome. Note masklike face and eye involvement.

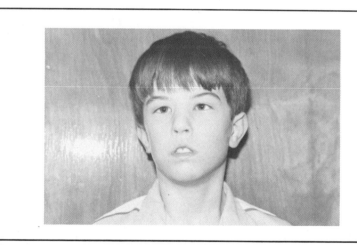

FIGURE 3-4.
Same boy at age 8. Cupid's bow of upper lip is shortened. Upper and lower lips do not meet in the midline.

Case Report

Michael came to the WMU Speech, Language and Hearing Clinic at the age of 2 years, 5 months with the diagnosis of Möbius syndrome. At birth Michael had severely clubbed feet and crossed eyes, and both conditions had been corrected surgically. He had characteristic involvement of the lateral rectus muscle so that he could move his eyes up and down but not laterally. He could not close his eyelids voluntarily, but when he was asleep, his eyelids closed involuntarily.

Michael had a high arched palate but no evidence of cleft. His gag reflex was active, and he had tactile sensation in his lips and face. He had experienced difficulty with bottle feeding. It had been necessary to squeeze his lips to form a circle that enabled him to suck. Occlusion was within normal limits. Bilateral tongue movements were slow, but he had no difficulty with tongue movements for articulation. His mouth was held open habitually. His face was typically masklike with no expression, which belied his intelligence. He expressed emotions by laughing or crying, but there was no smile or frown. He had repeated otitis media and a mild, intermittent conductive hearing loss. Articulation testing revealed difficulty with labial phonemes only. Michael was frustrated by attempts to close his lips for articulation and used his finger to push his lower lip up or his upper lip down to attain closure. He substituted /t, d/ for /p, b, m/.

Speech therapy focused on teaching Michael compensatory ways to produce bilabial sounds. Michael could move his articulators easily into the correct position for the /f/ and /v/ phonemes. Perceptually correct /p/ and /b/ sounds could be made by substituting the upper incisors for the upper lip with a buildup and sudden release of air pressure for the plosive feature. These compensatory sounds were taught like any new sounds. They were demonstrated in isolation, put into syllables, and then into words to substitute for /p, b, m/. Michael learned this production very quickly and advanced to word level in two therapy sessions.

Michael was a verbal and personable child who also learned compensations for his lack of facial expressions. He expressed his feelings verbally by saying, "I'm so happy." or "I'm smiling inside." He laughed when other children might smile. At age 8, he was doing accelerated work in a regular classroom at school and was happy and well adjusted. He does not receive speech therapy. Michael's case was uncomplicated due to his intelligence and isolated problem. Other children with Möbius syndrome may need extensive therapy.

Cornelia de Lange Syndrome

Children with Cornelia de Lange syndrome have an atypical masklike face with a small nose; thin, down-turned mouth; eyebrows that meet at the midline; and long, curly eyelashes. They also exhibit low birth weight; small stature; and increased body hair. Behavior disorders are reported in most cases, including self-mutilation. The incidence rate is 1 in 10,000 births and is thought to be a sporadic occurrence (Smith, 1982). The recurrence rate is 4% for the proband's siblings. No children are known to have been born to those with Cornelia de Lange syndrome.

Mental retardation is reported in all cases, usually accompanied by significant hearing loss and consistent severe language delay (Moore, 1970). An unusual birth cry is noted that could be described as a glottal fry: gutteral, feeble, and low pitched. Older children are capable of a range of higher vocal pitches, but their voices are habitually hoarse. Fraser and Campbell (1978) noted that the glottal fry continued in the children who did not develop speech. In those who did have useful language, the fry changed to hoarseness. Abnormalities in the speech structures are many and variable but do not account for the speech and voice dysfunction. There is marked individual variation in types and severity of the symptoms, but there are no reports of speech or language characteristics inconsistent with retardation or hearing loss other than the characteristic voice.

Noonan Syndrome

With an incidence of 1 in approximately 1,000 births, Noonan syndrome ranks among the more frequent disorders with multiple congenital anomalies. Etiology is sporadic (Smith, 1982). There is a great deal of variability of expression among patients with this diagnosis. It has been called the male Turner syndrome because of the phenotype of short stature, webbed neck, heart defects, skeletal abnormalities, and genital malformations, but it can occur in females as well. The general differences between Noonan and Turner syndromes are that there is more likely to be mental retardation in Noonan syndrome, and the congenital heart disease is more common and of a different type than in Turner syndrome. Frequent oral-facial characteristics are ptosis of the eyelids; strabismus; and flat, low nasal bridge. Auricles are sometimes low set or abnormal. Clefts of the uvula, high arched palate, and anterior dental malocclusion have also been reported (Hopkins-Acos & Bunker, 1979).

There is only one study of speech and hearing of several children with Noonan syndrome (Nora, Nora, Sinha, Spangler, & Lubs, 1974). Of 25 subjects, 72% had an articulation deficiency, and 12% had hearing difficulties. Unfortunately, there was no description of the difficulties or the evaluation instruments used.

Hopkins-Acos and Bunker (1979) report a clinical profile of speech and language in a child with Noonan syndrome before and after two years of speech therapy. He had a mild conductive hearing loss and had undergone extensive surgery for atrial septal defect and pulmonary stenosis. Formal assessment prior to therapy at age 3 years, 6 months on the Assessment of Children's Language Comprehension (ACLC) revealed that he was functioning significantly below age level in each subtest. He was also 1 to 1 1/2 years delayed in fine and gross motor skills. His expressive language consisted of gestures accompanied by nondistinguished utterances. No imitations could be elicited. Verbal output in the testing situation consisted of vowel sounds, laughter, and screaming. Treatment goals centered on improvement of fine and gross motor skills, turn taking, and speech in a functional communicative setting. Structured turn-taking activities required a response for continuation of activities. At first only motor responses were required, progressing to spontaneous imitation of peers' motor activities, and verbal imitation; then spontaneous verbal productions were required to continue an activity.

Reevaluation after 2 years of therapy indicated increased comprehension of two critical elements, but comprehension of three and four critical elements remained below norms. In conversational speech he used two and three elements per semantic utterance, but his speech remained unintelligible due to articulation differences. He had a consistent pattern of nasal substitutions for stop plosives, fricatives, sibilants, and glides in initial position.

The authors attribute the delay in language development in this case to limited sensory-motor experience due to his heart defect rather than to mental retardation. (Parental permission to obtain IQ scores could not be obtained.) He was placed in a normal kindergarten at 5 years, 11 months. By the end of the year, his skill levels were adequate except for the perceptual motor area where he had difficulty with a pencil or crayon, balancing on one foot, or throwing a ball. These perceptual motor differences, in addition to the mild hearing loss, were thought to be significant factors in relation to the child's language and phonological development.

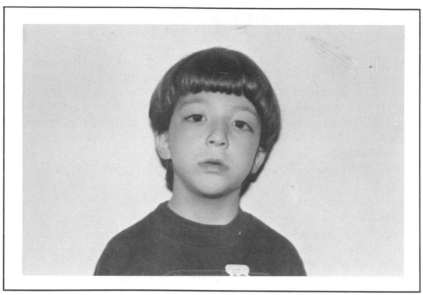

FIGURE 3-5.
Five-year-old boy with Noonan syndrome. Note wide nasal bridge, antimongoloid position of the eyes, and epicanthic folds.

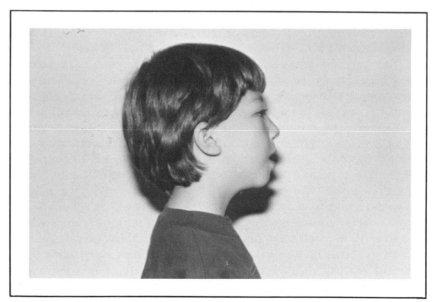

FIGURE 3-6.
Ears are rotated and low set in this child with Noonan syndrome.

Case Report

Tim weighed 8 lb, 4 oz at birth and required respiratory assistance to initiate breathing. During the pregnancy, his mother developed gestational diabetes, which was resolved following the birth. The parents became aware of developmental problems when Tim was 4 months old. He did not seem to localize sounds and did not roll over. At 15 months a chromosome study was done to rule out Down syndrome because of concern over the shape of his eyes and an overall developmental delay of approximately 4 months. The karyotype was normal. Tim developed five true words before he began to walk at 15 months. When walking began, the words ceased and were replaced by vowel sounds with inflectional change. At age 2 years, 9 months, he was evaluated at a parent-infant center. He was noted to have a very short attention span and had age-appropriate social skills, with mild to moderate delays in the area of fine motor, gross motor, and receptive language skills. On a subtest where he was asked to draw, the pencil had to be placed in his hand. A severe delay was evident in expressive language (7 to 9 month level). Therapy was begun to improve Tim's attention span and eye contact and was similiar to the imitative strategies outlined by Hopkins-Acos and Bunker (1979). Activities were first demonstrated by the clinician, then by the mother, and then Tim imitated. His eye contact and attention were reported to improve with this technique.

At age 3, Tim was evaluated at a genetics clinic and the diagnosis of Noonan syndrome was made by a pediatrician. Tim was in the 25th percentile for weight, 5th percentile for height, and 2nd percentile for head circumference. Physical examination noted excessively folded auricular helices, low-set ears, hypertelorism, inner epicanthic folds, downslant of palpebral fissures, high-arched palate, malocclusion, low posterior hairline, short broad neck, wide spaced nipples, and simian crease on both palms. He had a heart murmur consistent with ventricular septal defect.

At age 3 1/2, Tim was placed in a special education classroom that provided structured language activities plus speech therapy and occupational therapy for gross motor skills, balance, and coordination. He was using two- and three- word utterances with some echolalia. His language was telegraphic but functional. He had particular difficulty with initial consonant sounds. He was referred to an oral cleft clinic because of hypernasality and an unusual soft palate. Examination revealed a posterior pillar attachment that did not seem to function well during phonation. The plastic surgeon reported that it was likely that he was leaking air into the velopharyngeal area during spontaneous speech.

At age 5, he is approximately 1 year delayed in motor skills. He has not acquired a parachute reflex (extension of hands for protection) or hand preference. His hands, wrists, and face are hypotonic. Interestingly, like the child in the previous case, (Hopkins-Acos & Bunker, 1979), he cannot balance on one foot or throw a ball. Drooling has been a consistent problem. His height and weight are at the 50th percentiles for his age, but his head circumference remains at the 2nd percentile. On the Test of Oral Language Development (TOLD-P), Tim was approximately 2 years delayed in most language areas. Picture and oral vocabulary subtests had the most depressed scores. Placement and constriction errors were exhibited in multiple phoneme errors, but nearly all sounds could be produced in isolation. A mixture of hyponasality and hypernasality was noted. He has had recurrent ear infections and has had tubes placed in his ears twice. Some sensorineural hearing loss for high frequencies is evident. If the loss progresses, amplification will be necessary.

The single case study by Hopkins-Acos and Bunker (1979) was sufficiently detailed to allow comparison with Tim. Although conclusions cannot be drawn from profiles of just two cases, some striking similarities exist between these two boys: (a) hypernasality in the absence of cleft; (b) particular articulation difficulty with phonemes in the initial position; (c) mild hearing loss; (d) delay of 1 year in motor skills, specifically inability to balance on one foot and throw a ball; (e) prelinguistic problems with attention span and imitative behavior; (f) vocalizations of isolated vowel sounds from ages 2 to 3; and (g) therapy techniques directed at imitative interactive behavior. (There was no communication between anyone treating these independent cases.) A noteworthy difference in the cases is that Tim had a heart murmur but did not have surgery and the extended recovery period that the previous case experienced. While Hopkins-Acos and Bunker attribute the perceptual difficulties in their case to limited experience due to the heart problem, Tim did not have limited mobility and still exhibited similar problems. Perceptual-motor differences in addition to the mild hearing loss may certainly be significant factors in language and phonological development in Noonan syndrome. However, the cause of the perceptual-motor problem may be a part of the syndrome rather than a result of limited experiences.

Mental retardation may also be the cause, and it is unfortunate that IQ scores are not available for either case. It is hoped that clinicians who treat patients with Noonan syndrome will contribute case profiles including IQ data. The importance of early diagnosis must be stressed for subsequent referrals to an audiologist, speech clinician, and occupational therapist or physical therapist for intervention.

Table 3-2 describes speech and language in other disorders that are more rare than those in the previous discussion. The reader is referred to Siegel-Sadewitz and Shprintzen (1982) for the presence of speech signs in other syndromes.

NAME OF SYNDROME	PHYSICAL FEATURES	INHERITANCE PATTERN INCIDENCE RATE	SPEECH AND LANGUAGE CHARACTERISTICS	REFERENCES
Bloom Syndrome	Microcephaly; micrognathia; flared ears; eyelashes commonly lost; thin narrow face; marked sensitivity to sunlight	Autosomal recessive Half of patients are of Jewish descent 65 cases reported	High-pitched voice	Sedano, Sauk & Gorlin, 1977
Cutis Laxa	Skin hanging in loose folds; downward falling of both lips; accentuation of labial and labial medial sulci; micrognathia; abnormal tooth eruption	Severe autosomal recessive Benign autosomal dominant Rare X-linked form 50 cases reported	Hoarse cry from birth; unusually deep and resonant voice due to laxity in vocal cords	Sedano et al., 1977
Dubowitz Syndrome	Small head size, high receding forehead; flat supraorbital ridges; hypertelorism; micrognathia; sparse scalp hair and eyebrows; chronic rhinorrhea and serous otitis media; mild to moderate mental retardation with tendency toward hyperactivity and stubborness	Autosomal recessive Few cases reported	High-pitched weak cry; short attention span; high-pitched voice	Smith, 1982

TABLE 3-2
From "Speech and Language Characteristics of Genetic Syndromes," by S. Sparks and S. Millard, *Journal of Communication Disorders*, 1981, 14, pp. 411-419.

NAME OF SYNDROME	PHYSICAL FEATURES	INHERITANCE PATTERN INCIDENCE RATE	SPEECH AND LANGUAGE CHARACTERISTICS	REFERENCES
Familial Dysautonomia	Congenital indifference to pain; absence of tears; hypotension/hypertension; absence of lingual fungiform papillae; abnormal swallowing reflex; Episodic vomiting; erratic temperature control; poor motor coordination; absent or hypoactive deep tendon reflexes	Autosomal recessive Almost all parents are of Ashkenazi Jewish ancestry 1 in 10,000 to 1 in 20,000 births	Phoneme distortion; dysarthria; drooling; nasal, monotonous, slurred speech; lack of loudness control; normal receptive language	Sedano et al., 1977 Halpern, Hockberg, & Rees, 1967
Freeman-Sheldon Syndrome	Full forehead, mask-like face; small mouth-gives the appearance of whistling; deep set eyes; broad nasal bridge; small nose; long philtrum; H-shaped cutaneous dimpling on chin; Asymmetrical protruding ears; high palate; small tongue	Autosomal dominant very rare	Limited palatal movement with unclear nasal speech	Smith, 1982
Laurence-Moon-Biedl Syndrome	Retinitis pigmentosa; obesity; polydactyly; mental retardation; bifid uvula; high arched palate; moon-shaped face; varying degrees of microgenia	Autosomal recessive 1 in 60,000 live births	Varying articulation disorders; poor voluntary tongue and lip control; hypernasality; low vocal intensity; retarded language development; varying degrees of hearing impairment	Garstecki, Borton, Stark, & Kennedy, 1972

TABLE 3-2 (continued)

NAME OF SYNDROME	PHYSICAL FEATURES	INHERITANCE PATTERN INCIDENCE RATE	SPEECH AND LANGUAGE CHARACTERISTICS	REFERENCES
Mulibrey Nanism	Hydrocephalic skull; bulging forehead with prominent veins; triangular face; low nasal bridge; hypertelorism; reduced luster of retina-scarce pigmentation with dispersion and clusters of pigment	Autosomal recessive Prevalent in middle and eastern parts of Southern Finland	Weak, slightly hoarse, high-pitched voice; slight or moderate dysarthria	Goodman & Gorlin, 1977
Schwartz—Jampel Syndrome	Small face with sad, fixed facial appearance; long eyelashes in irregular rows; skeletal deformities; normal cognition; myopia	Autosomal recessive	High-pitched voice; drooling; indistinct speech; small mouth; puckered lips	Goodman & Gorlin, 1977 Bergsma, 1979
Ushers Syndrome	Congenital sensorineural hearing loss; retinitis pigmentosa, with cataracts; vestibular ataxia	Autosomal recessive 100% penetrance 1 in 20,000 1 in 80 are carriers	Variation from normal speech to characteristic deaf speech; may have congenital language pathology over and above that due to deafness	Vernon, 1969
Werner Syndrome	Short stature; loss of subcutaneous fat; pinched face with beak nose; gray sparse hair; retinal degeneration	Autosomal recessive 130 cases	High-pitched voice due to fibrous thickening in submucosal tissue	Goodman & Gorlin, 1977

TABLE 3-2 (continued)

REFERENCES

Apgar, V., & Beck, J. *Is my baby alright?* New York: Trident Press, 1972.

Azimov, I. *The genetic code.* New York: Orion Press, 1962.

Bedrossian, E.H., & Lachman, B.E. Congenital paralysis of the sixth and seventh cranial nerves: Congenital facial diplegia, congenital occulofacial palsy, Möbius syndrome. *American Journal of Ophthalmology,* 1956, *41,* 304-307.

Bergsma, D., (Ed.). *Birth defects compendium* (2nd ed.). New York: Liss, 1979.

Bergstrom, L. Causes of severe hearing loss in early childhood. *Pediatric Annals,* 1980, 9(1), 23-27.

Elfenbein, J., Waziri, M., & Morris, H.L. Verbal communication skills in six children with craniofacial anomalies. *Cleft Palate Journal,* 1981, 18(1), 59-64.

Fraser, W.I., & Campbell, B.M. A study of six cases of de Lange Amsterdam dwarf syndrome, with special attention to voice, speech and language characteristics. *Developmental Medicine and Child Neurology,* 1978, *20,* 189-198.

Garstecki, D.C., Borton, T.E., Stark, E.W., & Kennedy, B.T. Speech, language and hearing problems in Laurence-Moon-Biedl syndrome. *Journal of Speech and Hearing Disorders,* 1972, *37,* 407-413.

Genetic counseling and the prevention of Huntington's chorea. *Lancet,* 1982, *1,* 147.

Glass, L., Knapp, J., & Bloomer, H.H. Speech and lingual behavior before and after mandibular osteotomy. *Journal of Oral Surgery,* 1977, *35,* 104-109.

Glass, L., Stewart, R..E., & Miles, J. The speech-language pathologist's role in understanding the genetics of Van der Woude syndrome. *Journal of Speech and Hearing Disorders,* 1979, 44(4), 472-478.

Goodman, R.M., & Gorlin, R.J. *Atlas of the face in genetic disorders.* St. Louis: Mosby, 1977.

Gorlin, R.J., & Pindborg, J.J. Möbius syndrome. *Syndromes of the Head and Neck* (Chap. 74). New York: McGraw-Hill, 1964.

Halpern, H., Hockberg, I., & Rees, N. Speech and hearing characteristics of familial dysautonomia. *Journal of Speech and Hearing Research,* 1967, *10,* 361-366.

Hayes, E., Babin, R., & Platz, C. The otologic manifestations of mucopolysaccharidoses. *American Journal of Otology,* 1980, 2(2), 65-69.

Helmick, J.W. Speech characteristics of two children with Möbius syndrome. *Journal of Childhood Communication Disorders,* 1980, 4(1), 19-28.

Hopkins-Acos, P., & Bunker, K. A child with Noonan syndrome. *Journal of Speech and Hearing Disorders,* 1979, 44(4), 494-503.

Johnston, C. Taussig, L.M., Koopman, C., Smith, P., & Bjelland, J. Obstructive sleep apnea in Treacher-Collins syndrome. *Cleft Palate Journal,* 1981, 18(1), 39-44.

Kahane, J.C. Pathophysiological effects of Möbius syndrome on speech and hearing. *Archives of Otolaryngology,* 1979, 105(1), 29-34.

Karagan, N.J., & Zellweger, H.U. Early verbal disability in children with Duchenne muscular dystrophy. *Developmental Medicine and Child Neurology*, 1978, 20, 435-441.

Marsh, G.G., & Munsat, T.L. Evidence of early impairment of verbal intelligence in Duchenne muscular dystrophy. *Archives of Disease of Childhood*, 1974, 49, 118-122.

McKusick, V. *Medelian inheritance in man* (5th ed.). Baltimore: Johns Hopkins University Press, 1978.

Milunsky. A. *Know your genes*, Boston: Houghton-Mifflin, 1977.

Moore, M.V. Speech, hearing and language in de Lange syndrome. *Journal of Speech and Hearing Disorders*, 1970, 35, 66-69.

MPS Society brochure. (Available from the MPS Society, Inc., 552 Central Avenue, Bethpage, NY 11714.)

Nadler, H.L. Prenatal diagnosis of inborn defects: A status report. *Hospital Practice*, 1975, 10(66). (March of Dimes Reprint Series).

National Institutes of Health. *Huntington's disease: Hope through research* (publication no. 80-49). Bethesda, MD: National Institute of Neurological and Communicative Disorders and Stroke, October 1979.

Nora, J.J., Nora, A.H., Sinha, A.K., Spangler, R.D. & Lubs, H.A. The Ulrich Noonan syndrome (Turner phenotype). *American Journal of Diseases of Children*, 1974, 127, 48-55.

Peterson, S.J. Speech pathology in craniofacial malformations other than cleft lip and palate. *Proceedings of the Conference on Orofacial Anomalies: Clinical and Research Implications*, (ASHA Reports No. 8, pp. 111-131), August 1973.

Sedano, H.O., Sauk, J.J., & Gorlin, R.J. *Oral manifestations of inherited disorders*. Boston: Butterworth, 1977.

Shoulson, I., & Fahn, S. Huntington disease: Clinical care and evaluation. *Neurology*, 1979, 29, 1-3.

Siegel - Sadewitz, V., & Shprintzen, R.J. The relationship of communication disorders to syndrome identification. *Journal of Speech and Hearing Disorders*, 1982, 47(4), 338-345.

Smith, D.W. *Recognizable patterns of human malformation* (3rd ed.). Philadelphia: Saunders, 1982.

Sparks, S., & Millard, S. Speech and language characteristics of genetic syndromes. *Journal of Communication Disorders*, 1981, 14, 411-419.

Summer, G.K., & Shoaf, C.R. Developments in genetic and metabolic screening. *Family and Community Health*, 1982, 4(4), 13-29.

Thompson, J.S., & Thompson, M.W. *Genetics in medicine* (3rd ed.). Philadelphia: Saunders, 1980.

Vernon, M. Usher's syndrome: Deafness and progressive blindness. Clinical cases. *Journal of Chronic Diseases*, 1969, 22, 133-151.

Warkany, J. Craneostenosis. In J. Warkany, R.J. Lemire, & M.M. Cohen, Jr. (Eds.), *Mental retardation and congenital malformations of the central nervous system* (chap. 5). Chicago: Year Book Medical, 1981.

Witkop, C.J., & Henry, F.V. Sjogren-Larsson syndrome and histidinemia, hereditary biochemical diseases with defects of speech and oral functions. *Journal of Speech and Hearing Disorders*, 1963, *28*, 109-123.

Witzel, M.A., Ross, R.B., & Munro, I.R. Articulation before and after facial osteotomy. *Journal of Maxillofacial Surgery*, 1980, 8(3), 161-256.

Young, I.D., & Harper, P.D. Psychosocial problems in Hunter's syndrome. *Child: Care, Health and Development*, 1981, *7*, 201-209.

4

Multifactorial Genetic Disorders

Multifactorial traits reflect the combined effects of genetic factors acting in concert with prenatal environmental factors. It is believed that the majority of congenital disorders result from the interaction of genes and the intrauterine environment, but practically nothing is known about the nature of this interaction, which is infinitely varied (Ajl, 1982; Pernoll, King, & Prescott, 1980; Thompson & Thompson, 1980). The term "polygenic" is often used interchangeably with multifactorial, but polygenic should be reserved for those conditions in which a large number of genes act together without environment as a factor.

The pattern of occurrence in multifactorial disorders is clearly not Mendelian, because the recurrence rates are much lower than for single-gene disorders and distinct pedigrees cannot be constructed. Empirical risk data for these disorders, based on large statistical surveys, are scattered in the medical literature. For most multifactorial disorders the recurrence risk is usually 2 to 5% for first-degree relatives (parents, offspring, siblings) and less for second-degree relatives (aunts, nephews) and third-degree relatives (Bennett, 1981). Furthermore, the risk of occurrence of a trait depends upon an individual's susceptibility, or *threshold*, for that trait. (Threshold is discussed in more detail in the section on clefting in this chapter and in the section on teratogens in Chapter 5.) Criteria for multifactorial disorders are: (Bennett, 1981)

1. The trait occurs more often in relatives than in the general population. The risk to relatives declines with increasingly remote degrees of relationship.
2. The threshold effect may be lower in one sex, causing an imbalance in the frequency of affected individuals for one sex.

3. Studies of twins show a higher frequency of concordance (both twins have the trait) for monozygotic (identical) than for dizygotic (fraternal) twins.

4. The more severe the malformation, the higher the recurrence rate.

The limits of space do not allow discussion of all anomalies with multifactorial etiology, but for purposes of surveying speech disorders due to birth defects, three are of particular interest to clinicians. The multifactorial threshold has received wide support as an explanation of the etiology of cleft lip and palate and of neural tube defects and has been suggested as an explanation for stuttering, although it is highly controversial.

CLEFTING

Cleft lip and cleft palate are common birth defects occurring alone or in combination with other malformations in approximately 1.36 per 1,000 live births (Golbus, 1980). There are two individual cleft entities, recognized by all recent investigators, that are genetically and developmentally different. It is therefore important that cleft lip, with or without cleft palate CL(P), be distinguished from isolated cleft palate (CP). The complex nature of these two events must further be divided into two categories: syndromic, in which the clefting is one of several dysmorphic symptoms of a syndrome; and nonsyndromic, including (a) familial CL(P) and (b) nonfamilial, or isolated, CL(P) and CP (Fraser, 1970; Shields, Bixler, & Fogh-Andersen, 1981).

Syndromic Clefting

Cohen (1978) identified 154 syndromes that included cleft lip and cleft palate, twice as many as were identified in 1971. Of these, 29 are chromosomal, and 79 are single-gene disorders (autosomal dominant, 35; autosomal recessive, 39; and X-linked, 5). Syndrome identification, including syndromes with clefting, is an ongoing process, and undoubtedly many more syndromes will be delineated in the future. The risk of occurrence for clefting is the same as for the occurrence of the syndrome. The remaining syndromes with clefting may be sporadic in etiology, such as in femoral hypoplasia-unusual facies syndrome, or they may have specific environmental causes, as in fetal alcohol syndrome. For a comprehensive discussion of clefting in syndromes, see Smith (1982) and Cohen (1978).

The following case reports are illustrations of rare syndromes in which severe clefts are among the features of the syndrome. Both children have made reasonable accommodation to their disability. Although both syndromes are sporadic (nongenetic), the first case poses some unique problems because of other disorders in the family that are genetic. In the second case, speech was considerably better after surgery than in the first, so much so that speech therapy was not required. So little is known about these syndromes that it is impossible to know if these children are typical. Cases such as these should receive the services of an oral-cleft team and a genetic counselor.

Case Report

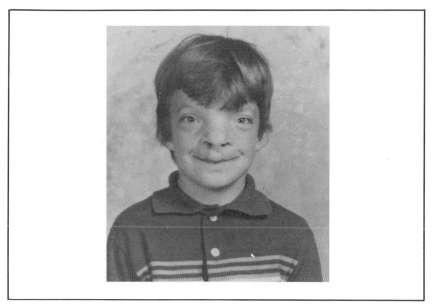

FIGURE 4-1
Child with medial cleft face syndrome. Note extent of hypertelorism.

Jason is a 6-year-old boy with a syndromic bilateral cleft lip and palate that extended to his nose, called *medial cleft face syndrome with hypertelorism*. This disorder may be mistaken for *medial cleft lip syndrome*, a disorder that has a poor prognosis, including mental retardation and limited survival. In contrast, medial cleft face syndrome probands usually have normal intelligence and life expectancy (Fraser, 1971).

Jason's father was in the delivery room when he was born and was aware immediately that his son had a cleft lip. According to the father, the parents received little help because their physician and the hospital personnel did not know how to deal with the child's problem. His father fed Jason with a shot glass because he was unable to suck. Attempts to place an endotracheal tube were fought off by the infant. Jason was referred to a cleft palate team, which included a plastic surgeon, speech pathologist, audiologist, otolaryngologist, psychologist, orthodontist, educational specialist, and genetic counselor. A series of surgical procedures was undertaken: lip closure at 2 months, soft palate repair at 2 years, cosmetic lip surgery at 3 years, myringotomies at ages 4 and 5, hard palate repair at age 5 that reopened soon after, and a pharyngeal flap at age 6. Prior to the pharyngeal flap surgery, he had frequent colds and ear infections.

Medial cleft face syndrome is usually sporadic but has some features that are similar to chromosomal, autosomal dominant, and polygenic syndromes. Jason's karyotype revealed no chromosomal defects, and the suspected autosomal dominant disorders were eliminated by physical examination. There was no known family history of clefting or congenital facial abnormalities in his mother's history. His father had been adopted and no family history was available. Jason's syndrome is most likely sporadic with little risk of recurrence in other offspring of these parents. However, Jason's own children have a 50% chance of inheritance of the anomaly.

The genetic counselor found that this child is at risk for a number of complications arising from a complex genetic history. His father has neurofibromatosis, an autosomal dominant disorder resulting in tumors on the body arising from neural tissue (Riccardi, 1981). Jason's mother had lost an eye at age 2 to retinoblastoma, a cancer regarded as a birth defect and linked to a threshold of susceptibility from genetic and environmental factors (Decker & Goldstein, 1982; Gerald, 1979). Jason's parents adopted their first two children because they feared that their problems might be transmitted genetically but then elected to have Jason and his sister, who is normal. Jason and his sister, therefore, have a 50% chance of neurofibromatosis and may have a genetic susceptibility to retinoblastoma. An environmental factor that could complicate the latter disorder is radiation. Jason's parents were counseled to avoid X-rays of Jason's head and neck in future plans for surgery and orthodontia. This was very important advice that might have been missed without the services of a geneticist as part of the team of professionals who evaluated the child.

Jason is distractible in school, and his speech is sometimes unintelligible due to hypernasality and multiple articulation problems. In spite of this, Jason is outgoing, friendly, and has many friends. A value system of tolerance and acceptance of differences is apparent in this home. The father made it clear that the word "handicapped" is not so much a physical concept as a way of looking at the world (Multiclinic 49, 1980).

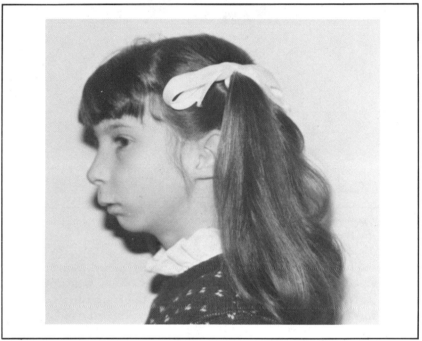

FIGURE 4-2
Eleven-year-old girl with femoral hydroplasia-unusual facies syndrome (FH-UFS). Note micrognathia and broad, flattened tip of nose.

Case Report

Mary was born with absent femurs (thigh bones), absent labia majora, clefts of the soft and hard palates, and an atypical face, which led to the diagnosis of *femoral hypoplasia-unusual facies syndrome* (FH-UFS). Her normal tibias were attached directly to her pelvis (Hurst & Johnson, 1980). This sporadic syndrome has also been described as bilateral femoral dysgenesis syndrome. Figures 4-2 and 4-3 illustrate her facial characteristics of upslanting palpebral fissures, short nose, broad nasal tip, long philtrum, and micrognathia. These signs constitute a pattern of dysmorphology, as outlined in Chapter 1. A few cases of this rare syn-

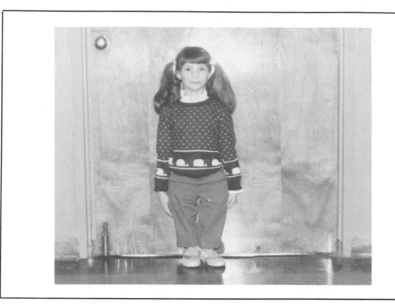

FIGURE 4-3
Same girl with FH-UFS. Femurs are absent.

drome have been reported in the literature (Daentl, Smith, Scott, Hall, & Gooding, 1975; Goldberg, Fish, Cohen, & Shprintzen, 1978). Intelligence was normal in all affected individuals.

Her mother was 28 and her father was 27 at the time of her birth. She weighed 4 lb and 7 oz, was 14 in. long, and was full term. There was no family history of birth defects. At 5 weeks into the pregnancy, the mother was given a progestational agent as a pregnancy test. No other drugs were taken early in the pregnancy. The father had been exposed to Agent Orange, a possible teratogen currently under investigation. At age 1, Mary had surgery to close two thirds of the soft palate. She began to use single words at that time, but hypernasality and multiple articulation errors made her speech unintelligible. Her receptive skills were not impaired. She began speech therapy at the WMU Speech, Language and Hearing Clinic at age 2. Speech goals followed traditional lines for a young patient with cleft palate. Therapy focused on correct placement of the articulators for phonemes; she had devised her own system of compensatory placements, such as glottal stops and nasal snorts for plosive sounds. Her lingual frenulum was too short for her tongue tip to reach the alveolar ridge, and it was clipped at age 2 1/2. At age 4, Mary had pharyngeal flap surgery. The goal of speech therapy after surgery was to maintain the previously learned articulation placements and to integrate them into her spontaneous speech. Mary corrected her articulation errors quickly after the pharyngeal flap controlled the nasal emission of air during speech.

Although her parents had been told at her birth that Mary would probably never walk, she sat at 8 months, stood at 12 months, and began to walk at 19 months by rotating her body from side to side. She wore 5-in. shoe lifts for height. She received occupational therapy where a special tricycle with hand controls was built for her. Mary's personality was characterized by independence. She insisted on doing whatever she could for herself. When she started to attend kindergarten, further speech therapy was not necessary. She has prostheses for her legs but prefers not to wear them. At age 11 she enjoys gymnastics and is well adjusted at school.

Nonsyndromic Clefting

Two factors complicate simple explanations for the etiology of those classifications of CP and CL(P) that are not symptoms of a syndrome: (a) etiological heterogeneity and (b) individual threshold of expression.

Etiological heterogeneity

Both CP and CL(P) are heterogeneous. That is, the phenotypes of CP and CL(P) can be caused by familial etiology or be an isolated event. Familial cases (two or more affected first-, second-, or third-degree relatives) comprise about 25% of all CL(P) occurrences and 12% of all CP occurrences. Isolated cases are heterogeneous and represent the largest group: 74% of CL(P) cases and 80% of CP cases (Bixler, 1981). There are significant differences between the familial and isolated etiology groups (Shields et al., 1981): (a) Increased incidence of isolated occurrences has been noted in particular years while the incidence of familial cases remains constant. (b) In familial cases, females are more severely affected than males. (c) The malformation rate for congenital defects other than clefts in the siblings of probands is five times higher in isolated cases than in the familial group, which suggests some predisposing factors in these families. This malformation rate is not increased in parents and other relatives. (d) In the isolated group, as the mother's age increases, so does the incidence of CP, but the relationship of maternal age to CP is not observed in the familial group.

Threshold of expression

This concept suggests that there is an underlying liability for a trait in each individual that encompasses both genetic and physiological factors. The cumulative effect of these genetic and physiological factors may or may not cross an individual's threshold of expression of that trait. For example, there is a prenatal developmental stage at which the palatal shelves become horizontal and flatten in order to fuse. Many factors, genetic and environmental, interact to determine when this occurs during fetal development. If it has not occurred by a certain stage of growth, the shelves will be unable to reach each other to fuse, and a cleft palate results. This stage can be considered a developmental threshold, distinguishing between normal fetuses and those that will have cleft palate. There are many ways in which the genetic and environmental factors can be altered to increase the probability that a fetus will fall below that developmental threshold. Genes that alter the shape of the face can cause increased head width, increased tongue size, reduced tongue mobility, reduced mandible growth, reduced shelf width, reduction of the force that causes the shelves to move, and so forth. The fetus with a susceptible face shape is near the developmental threshold, and slight retardation of growth of one of the processes could be enough to cause a cleft, whereas in the fetus with a resistant face shape, the same retardation would not cause a defect (Fraser, 1970, 1971). Additionally, some outside agents can be implicated in a small proportion of cases. The Center for Disease Control (Golbus, 1980) demonstrated that the relative risk for CL(P) in infants exposed to diazepam (Valium) during the first trimester of pregnancy was four-fold. There is also a suggested association of oral clefts from prenatal amphetamine exposure and of CL(P) among infants exposed to antiepileptic medication in utero (Golbus, 1980).

Obviously, predicting recurrence risk for clefts is exceedingly complex. Table 4-1 gives estimates of the risk of recurrence for various situations. It should be emphasized that these data reflect averages, and some families will have a higher or lower risk than those presented. For definitive information on recurrence, the inquiring family members should be referred for genetic counseling (see Chapter 7). Some of those cases thought to be nonsyndromic could, in fact, have escaped detection. Shields et al. (1981) suggest that a detailed medical examination of the proband for such subtle associated abnormalities as hyperkinesis, learning disability, and growth retardation may uncover a clefting malformation syndrome in individuals thought to be nonsyndromic. Geis, Seto, Bar-

Situation	Proband has CL ± CP	Proband has CP
Frequency of defect in the general population	0.1%	0.04%
My spouse and I are unaffected.		
1. We have an affected child.		
What is the probability that our next baby will have the same condition if:		
We have no affected relatives?	4%	2%
There is an affected relative?	4%	7%
Our affected child also has another malformation?	2%	2%
My spouse and I are related?	4%	—
What is the probability that our next baby will have some other sort of malformation?	Same as general population	Same as general population
2. We have two affected children.		
What is the probability that our next baby will have the same condition?	9%	1%
I am affected (or my spouse is).		
1. We have no affected children.		
What is the probability that our next baby will be affected?	4%	6%
2. We have an affected child.		
What is the probability that our next baby will be affected?	17%	15%

TABLE 4-1
Counseling risks for cleft lip with or without cleft palate (CL ± CP) and cleft palate (CP) for various situations. From "Etiology of Cleft Lip and Palate" by F.C. Fraser, In *Cleft Lip and Palate*, Little, Brown, 1971. Copyright by W.C. Grabb, S. Rosenstein, & K.R. Bzoch (Eds.). Reprinted by permission.

toshesky, Lewis, and Pashayan (1981) found a tenfold increase in the prevalence risk of congenital heart disease with clefting. Exclusive of Pierre-Robin anomalad and syndromic clefts, the highest prevalence of heart disease was in those children with bilateral CL(P). The lowest incidence of heart disease with clefting was in those patients with cleft lip only and no associated syndrome.

Pierre-Robin Anomalad

The Pierre-Robin anomalad is characterized by a U-shaped cleft palate; small, recessed lower jaw; and carriage of the tongue down and out of the mouth. Pierre-Robin anomalad is a phenotype found in a number of syndromes, such as trisomy 18. It can also be the result of multifactorial causation as a mechanical constraint prior to 9 weeks gestation in which the chin is compressed in such a manner that the tongue impairs the closure of the posterior palatal shelves that must grow to meet in the midline. Postnatally, the small jaw usually shows some improvement as the child grows older, and surgery to repair the jaw is usually delayed until some catching up in development has taken place (Smith, 1982). Feeding problems and upper airway obstruction that sometimes requires tracheostomy are of primary concern in the newborn with Pierre-Robin anomalad. Approximately 70% of the children with Pierre-Robin anomalad also have congenital conductive hearing loss (Bergstrom, 1980). All documented speech problems associated with this anomalad are characteristically due to hearing loss, the cleft condition, or the malocclusion (Bloomer, 1971).

STUTTERING

Any discussion of speech and language disorders with genetic etiology must address the recent speculation that stuttering has a genetic component. Stuttering does run in families, but, to date, no simple pattern of Mendelian inheritance has been shown to be compatible with pedigrees of stutterers, and no single gene locus has been identified. K.K. Kidd and his associates in the Department of Human Genetics at the Yale University School of Medicine have studied stuttering proband pedigrees extensively and found that stuttering does not follow a pattern of autosomal dominant, autosomal recessive, or sex-linked inheritance (Kidd, 1980; Kidd, Heimbuch, Records, Oehlert, & Webster, 1980; Records, K.K. Kidd, & J.R. Kidd, 1977). However, a number of methodological contraints may influence the quality of the data. Investigators of genetic etiologies for stuttering suggest that there are two distinct kinds of stuttering: that which is outgrown and that which persists into adulthood (Records et al., 1977; Sheehan & Costley, 1977). In family pedigrees of proband stutterers, it is likely that information about individuals who stuttered as children but recovered may be unreported or underreported. If a parent or sibling stuttered for only a short time at an early age, it may have been forgotten or never mentioned to the proband.

It is interesting to note how stuttering fits the criteria for multifactorial disorders at the beginning of this chapter. The evidence for multifactorial susceptibility with a threshold effect is intriguing and is presented here with the caution, prominent in all the studies cited, that the current evidence is insufficient to prove a hypothesis of genetic etiology.

Risk of occurrence

Stuttering does run in families. The proportion of stutterers who have a familial history of stuttering is about one fourth to one third (Andrews & Harris, 1964; Sheehan & Costly, 1977). If at least one parent, as opposed to a sibling, ever stuttered, the familial risk is significantly increased. If the proband is female, the familial risk is significantly increased again (Kidd, 1980). Andrews et al. (1983) pooled the data from 725 families covered by the Andrews and Harris (1964) and Kidd (1980) studies and estimated the following risks. For men who ever stuttered, 9% of their daughters and 22% of their sons will be stutterers. For women who ever stuttered, the risks are higher, as 17% of their daughters and 36% of their sons will be affected. The incidence figures are hard to explain on a purely cultural level, because incidence and prevalence figures are consistent in various populations and cultures (Goodall & Brobby, 1982). If stuttering were a purely cultural or learned phenomenon, more variation across cultures would be expected.

Sex ratio

The sex ratio of stuttering is approximately five males to one female (Records et al., 1977; Sheehan & Costly, 1977). This would suggest a predisposing factor connected with maleness. There are sufficient examples of father-to-son transmission to reject X-linked inheritance. If not X linked, the evidence of sex difference might be explained by a threshold theory; males have more than twice the risk of females. Whatever factors contribute to susceptibility to stuttering may be characterized by lower thresholds for males. Furthermore, if those factors were transmitted, female stutterers would transmit more factors, and the families of female stutterers would thus have more members who stutter. The incidence figures show that there are more stutterers in the families of female stutterers (Kidd et al., 1980). However, as Ferry, Culbertson, Fitzgibbons, and Netsky (1979) have pointed out, males are more susceptible to perinatal and prenatal environmental insult than are females and have higher incidences of autism, learning disabilities, and language problems in general. It is reasonable that the same vulnerability to nongenetic factors could also account for the sex ratio in stuttering.

Studies of twins

If there were a genetic predisposition, it would follow that the same susceptibility would occur in identical (monozygotic) twins. Studies have shown that monozygotic twins have a higher concordance for stuttering than do dizygotic same-sex twins. Andrews et al., (1983) estimate that a monozygotic co-twin has an estimated 77% chance of being a stutterer, a dizygotic same-sex co-twin has a 32% chance of being a stutterer, and a same-sex sibling has an 18% chance of being a stutterer. However, monozygotic twin pairs do exist who are discordant for stuttering (Howie, 1976, 1981). Andrews et al., (1983) conclude that pre- or postnatal environmental factors must be important to some stutterers. Such factors have been looked for in discordant monozygotic twins, but none have been identified.

Severity

Those individuals determined to be the most genetically predisposed are not the most severely affected; that is, those with the most first-degree relatives who ever stuttered are not the most severe stutterers (Kidd, 1980). If there is a genetic component to whether or not an individual ever stutters, that genetic component need not be related to severity.

Summary

Sheehan and Costley (1977) raise the possibility that the type of stuttering that occurs in childhood and has a spontaneous recovery by adolescence is a developmental disorder for some predisposed genotypes. Although the data are contradictory, there is enough evidence of genetic predisposition for stuttering to warrant further interest and investigation. As Harris (1977) notes: If by research, one could identify those who are genetically predisposed to a particular condition, one would have a powerful tool with which to discover the critical environmental factors. It would be possible to ask what major differences exist or have existed between the environmental circumstances of the predisposed persons and those in whom the condition does not develop. Therefore, if the environmental circumstances can be recognized, they can be modified for the genetically predisposed person before the stuttering develops. If there are persons genetically predisposed to stuttering, research must be directed to those environmental factors critical to the development of stuttering.

NEURAL TUBE DEFECTS

Neural tube defects are multifactorial birth defects in which part of the brain is absent (anencephaly) or the spinal cord is not covered with skin and bone (spina bifida). Most infants with anencephaly die soon after birth. Spina bifida is a developmental defect of the spinal column in which one or more spinal vertebral arches fail to fuse and in which the underlying spinal cord is damaged. There are various degrees of severity in spina bifida ranging from spina bifida occulta, in which the defect is in the bony arch only, to spina bifida aperta, often associated with meningocele (protrusion of the meninges) or meningomyelocele (protrusion of neural elements as well as meninges). In addition to the mass on the back, clinical features include hydrocephalus; locomotor paralysis; sensory and autonomic disturbances; bladder and bowel incontinence; and disturbances in mental and emotional development (Smith, 1982).

The recurrence rate of neural tube defects is 3% for first-degree, 1.2% for second-degree, and 0.5% for third-degree relatives. It is relatively common but has marked variation in incidence from one country to another. It occurs in 0.6 to 4.1 of 1,000 live births in the United States. The incidence is higher in girls than in boys. In recent years an increasing number of children with this defect are surviving longer (Colgan, 1981; Thompson & Thompson, 1980).

Spina Bifida

Spina bifida is an example of a birth defect involving multiple organ systems that requires complex medical, social, ethical, economic, and educational decisions. Many infants born with spina bifida are so severely abnormal that they do not survive, and others have minimal defects, but there is an intermediate group in which even if surgical intervention is successful, the child is left with partial or complete paresis of the lower limbs and fecal and urinary incontinence. When the condition is accompanied by hydrocephalus, the insertion of a ventricular-jugular-atrial shunt to relieve the accumulation of cerebrospinal fluid is often required.

Intelligence in spina bifida

Most children with meningomyelocele have IQs in the normal range. The likelihood of normal intelligence is highest for those children with low lesions and no hydrocephalus. However, there is a high probability of learning disability in these children, and preschool testing should be considered to avoid the possibility of educational failure because of lack of recognition of learning problems. It is of utmost importance that the use of the intellect be optimal and that the opportunity to experience success academically not be jeopardized. The upright position with hands free, is strongly recommended for a child to accomplish appropriate developmental tasks and for interaction with peers (Colgan, 1981).

Hydrocephalus

The intellectual potential is considerably different for those children with spina bifida who also have the complication of hydrocephalus. Dennis et al. (1981) studied the intelligence of 78 hydrocephalic children and uncovered some patterns that have clinical significance.

A common outcome of hydrocephalus is uneven cognitive growth during childhood, with nonverbal intelligence developing less fully than verbal intelligence. This behavior depends more on the concomitants of hydrocephalus than on the condition itself. certain etiological, biomechanical, and symptomatic aspects of the condition. Some abnormalities of brain development in the hydrocephalic child limit nonverbal intelligence.

Hydrocephalus thins and distends the brain. If treatment is instituted in the first months of life, hydrocephalus does not progressively debilitate intelligence throughout childhood. But some of the effects of hydrocephalus persist into childhood, even after successful treatment. Regional cortical thinning appears to be related directly to a particular pattern of intellectual development.

The features that lowered the absolute or relative levels of nonverbal intelligence in these children as a result of the hydrocephalus are impaired motor function, impaired visual function, and seizures. Hydrocephalus affects gross motor function by deforming the cerebellum; fine motor control by disturbing the kinesthetic-proprioceptive basis of hand control; and bimanual motor function by causing stretching of the corpus callosum. These impairments in fine motor control make it difficult for the hydrocephalic child to perform normally on time-limited nonverbal intelligence tasks. Ocular problems and seizures also were correlated with impaired nonverbal intelligence. The authors speculate that nonverbal intelligence may be more vulnerable than verbal intelligence to even a single early seizure.

The Cocktail Party Syndrome

A distinctive type of language known as the cocktail party syndrome (CPS) appears to be specific to some children with hydrocephalus. Taylor (1961) described these children as very sociable with an impressive verbal ability and a good memory for social occurrences and auditory series. However, their intellectual performance was limited by defective perceptual-motor skills and a lack of judgement, reasoning, and comprehension. They have been called "chatterers" with unusual verbal fluency. Their articulation is mature and precise. Even difficult polysyllabic words are well articulated. The children enjoy imitating words (Schwartz, 1974). The cocktail party syndrome should not be confused with echolalia, as the child is able to initiate dialogue.

Tew (1979) calls the cocktail party syndrome a combination of unusual verbal fluency coupled with certain personality characteristics. He studied 59 children, aged 5, who were hydrocephalic and had spina bifida. They were considered to have the syndrome if they had four of the following five criteria: (a) perseveration of response, either echoing the examiner or repetition of an earlier statement made by the child; (b) excessive use of social phrases in conversation; (c) over-familiarity in manner, not normally expected in a 5-year-old child; (d) habit of introducing personal experience into the conversation in irrelevent and inappropriate contexts; and (e) fluent and normally well-articulated speech.

The results of detailed psychological testing in this study by Tew (1979) showed that children with the cocktail party syndrome can be distinguished from other cases of spina bifida as having significantly lower Wechsler Intelligence Test scores and very retarded social skills. Visual perceptual abilities were also significantly poorer. The verbal fluency did not lead to superior scores on the Reynell Expressive Language Scales, for these children found difficulty in using language creatively in spite of good syntax. In fact, the expressive language scores were approximately 7 months below their scores on the language comprehension scale, and 2 1/2 years below their chronological age. Further assessment at the age of 7 revealed these children to be significantly poorer than other cases of spina bifida in reading, spelling, and arithmetic, and they had shorter attention spans and slightly more behavior problems in school. There was evidence that the cocktail party syndrome declines with age, and its presence at the age of 10 is diagnostically significant of a subnormal level of intelligence.

Whether the etiology of the cocktail party syndrome is a result of neuropathology or is due to selective reinforcement by adults is unknown. Visual defects were found in 65% of Tew's subjects, and they had more severe physical disability as a group than did the control group of spina bifida without CPS. Tew's results suggest that CPS is most likely to occur in severely disabled girls confined to wheelchairs, with valve-controlled hydrocephalus.

There is a suggestion that CPS is reinforced by parents. Jensen and Kogan (1962) have shown that the parents regard their handicapped child's conversation as evidence of normal intelligence. The emergence of language in a hydrocephalic spina bifida child may be a source of delight and comfort to the parents, and they believe that the intellect is unimpaired. The type of family who seems to be most likely to encourage CPS are described by Schaffer (1964) as inward looking with the child as the focus of an abnormal degree of attention from all members of the family.

Summary

The research concerning intelligence in spina bifida children and aberrant language patterns in children with hydrocephalus has implications for clinicians. Prior to the research of Dennis et al. (1981) and Tew (1979), Schwartz (1974) wrote that "the speech clinician's role in dealing with the child with myelomengocele is minimal, since the children, as a group, develop adequate language. Long term observation and evaluation show that the children follow a normal language progression . . . Although cocktail party speech is an interesting phenomenon not now understood, it requires little direct intervention on the part of the speech clinician" (pp. 465-467). On the contrary, the clinician should have an active role on the multidisciplinary rehabilitation team that these children require.

Speech and language testing for all children with spina bifida, even without signs of language disorder, is essential to discern any problems at the earliest possible stage. These children with physical problems must have optimal use of their language skills for maximum independence and psychosocial development. The clinician should be alert to the motor and visual problems that limit their interaction with their environment and may interfere with testing procedures.

The language of children with hydrocephalus in spina bifida has not received the attention it deserves. The fluent and precisely articulated speech may mask severe comprehension problems. Perhaps the most difficult task for the clinician may be to convince the parents that language problems can exist in their hydrocephalic child when that is the area in which they take pride. The parent should be helped to listen to the excesses in the child's speech and reinforce desired behaviors.

Tew (1979) recommends that treatment methods should not differ in principle from the conditioning procedures of other language disorders. This remains to be seen until published accounts of therapy are available.

REFERENCES

Ajl, S.J. Birth defects research: 1980 and after. *American Journal of Medicine*, 1982, 72, 119-126.

Andrews, G., Craig, A., Feyer, A.M., Hoddinott, S., Howie, P., & Neilson, M. Stuttering: A review of research findings and theories circa 1982. *Journal of Speech and Hearing Disorders*, 1983, 48(3), 226-246.

Andrews, G., & Harris, M. *The syndrome of stuttering.* London: Heinemann Books, 1964.

Bennett, J.W. A primer in human genetics. In K.I. Abroms & J.W. Bennett (Eds.), *Issues in genetics and exceptional children.* San Francisco: Jossey-Bass, 1981.

Bergstrom, L. Causes of severe hearing loss in early childhood. *Pediatric Annals*, 1980, 9(1), 23-27.

Bixler, D. Genetics and clefting. *Cleft Palate Journal*, 1981, 18(1), 10-18.

Bloomer, H.H. Speech defects associated with dental malocclusions and related abnormalities. In L.D. Travis (Ed.), *Handbook of speech pathology and audiology.* New York: Appleton-Century-Crofts, 1971.

Cohen, M.M. Syndromes with cleft lip and cleft palate. *Cleft Palate Journal*, 1978, 15(4), 306-325.

Colgan, M.T. The child with spina bifida. *American Journal of Diseases of Children*, 1981, 135, 854-858.

Daentl, D.L., Smith, D.W., Scott, C.I., Hall, B.D., & Gooding, C.A. Femoral hypoplasia-unusual facies syndrome. *The Journal of Pediatrics*, 1975, 86, 107-111.

Decker, J., & Goldstein, J.C. Risk factors in head and neck cancer. *New England Journal of Medicine*, 1982, 306(19), 151-1155.

Dennis, M., Fitz, C.R., Netley, C.T., Sugar, J., Harwood-Nash, D.C.F., Hendrick, A.B., Hoffman, H.J., & Humphreys, R.P. The intelligence of hydrocephalic children. *Archives of Neurology,* 1981, *38,* 605-615.

Ferry, P.C., Culbertson, J.L., Fitzgibbons, P.M., & Netsky, M.G. Brain function and language disabilities. *International Journal of Pediatric Otorhinolaryngology,* 1979, *1,* 13-24.

Fraser, F.C. The genetics of cleft lip and cleft palate. *American Journal of Human Genetics,* 1970, *22*(3), 336-352.

Fraser, F.C. Etiology of cleft lip and palate. In W.C. Grabb, S.W. Rosenstein, & K.R. Bzoch (Eds), *Cleft lip and palate* (pp. 54-65). Boston: Little, Brown, 1971.

Geis, N., Seto, B., Bartoshesky, L., Lewis, M.B., & Pashayan, H.M. The prevalence of congenital heart disease among the population of a metropolitan cleft lip and palate clinic. *Cleft Palate Journal,* 1981, *18*(1), 19-23.

Gerald, P.S. Chromosome analysis techniques expand: New links to cancer. *Journal of the American Medical Association,* 1979, *242*(12), 1239-1240.

Golbus, M.S. Teratology for the obstetrician: Current status. *Obstetrics and Gynecology,* 1980, *55*(3), 1-9.

Goldberg, R.B., Fish, B., Cohen, M.M., & Shprintzen, R.J. Bilateral femoral dysgenesis syndrome: A case report. *Cleft Palate Journal,* 1978, *15*(4), 386-389.

Goodall, H.B., & Brobby, G.W. Stuttering, sickling, and cerebral malaria: A possible organic basis for stuttering. *Lancet,* 1982, *1*(8284), 1279-1280.

Harris, H. Nature and nurture. *New England Journal of Medicine,* 1977, *297*(25), 1399-1400.

Howie, P.M. *A twin investigation of the etiology of stuttering.* Paper presented at the Annual Convention of the American Speech and Hearing Association, Houston, November 1976.

Howie, P.M. Concordance for stuttering in monozygotic and dizygotic twin pairs. *Journal of Speech and Hearing Research,* 1981, *24*(3), 317-321.

Hurst, D., & Johnson, D. Brief clinical report: Femoral hypoplasia-unusual facies syndrome. *American Journal of Medical Genetics,* 1980, *5,* 255-258.

Jensen, G.D., & Kogan, K.L. Parental estimates of the future achievement of cerebral palsied children. *Journal of Mental Deficiency Research,* 1962, *6,* 56.

Kidd, K.K. Genetic models of stuttering. *Journal of Fluency Disorders,* 1980, *5,* 187-201.

Kidd, K.K., Heimbuch, R.C., Records, M.A., Oehlert, G., & Webster, R.L. Familial stuttering patterns are not related to one measure of severity. *Journal of Speech and Hearing Research,* 1980, *23*(3), 539-545.

Multiclinic 49. Videotape presented at the College of Health & Human Services, Western Michigan University, January, 1980.

Pernoll, M.L., King, C.R., & Prescott, G.H. Genetics for the clinical obstetrician-gynecologist. *Obstetrics and Gynecology Annual,* 1980, *9,* 1-53.

Records, M.A., Kidd, K.K., & Kidd, J.R. *The family clustering of stuttering.* Paper presented at the Annual Convention of the American Speech and Hearing Association, Chicago, November, 1977.

Riccardi, M.M. Von Recklinhausen neurofibromatosis. *New England Journal of Medicine*, 1981, 35(27), 1617-1618.

Schaffer, H.R. The "too-cohesive" family. A form of group pathology. *International Journal of Social Psychiatry*, 1964, 10, 266.

Schwartz, E.R. Characteristics of speech and language development in the child with myelomeningocele and hydrocephalus. *Journal of Speech and Hearing Disorders*, 1974, 39, 465-468.

Sheehan, J.G., & Costley, M.S. A reexamination of the role of heredity in stuttering. *Journal of Speech and Hearing Disorders*, 1977, 42, 47-58.

Shields, E., Bixler, D., & Fogh-Andersen, P. Cleft palate: A genetic and epidemiologic investigation. *Clinical Genetics*, 1981, 20, 13-24.

Smith, D.W. *Recognizable patterns of human malformation* (3rd ed.). Philadelphia: Saunders, 1982.

Taylor, E.M. *Psychological appraisal of children with cerebral deficits.* Cambridge, MA: Harvard University Press, 1961.

Tew, B. The "cocktail party syndrome" in children with hydrocephalus and spina bifida. *British Journal of Disorders of Communication*, 1979, 14, 85-101.

Thompson, J.S. & Thompson, M.W. *Genetics in medicine* (3rd ed.). Philadelphia: Saunders, 1980.

5

Environmental
Birth Defects

Environmental causes of birth defects are those that act upon the developing fetus in the environment of the uterus after the genetic coding has taken place. The causes of secondary growth deficiency originate outside the fetus and limit its capacity for growth. Differentiating genetic from nongenetic origins of congenital defects is not easy, however, because many birth defects are suspected to arise from the genetic susceptibility of the fetus to an environmental insult. Some children may be severely affected with very little exposure to a prenatal insult, and some may not be affected after large amounts of exposure.

This chapter will discuss fetal malnutrition, teratogens (agents that cause fetal malformations), and diseases— the major causes of insult resulting in secondary growth deficiency that may have an effect on brain development and, in turn, on cognition, oromuscular development, language, and speech of the affected child. The clinician who deals with the diagnosis of environmental (and therefore preventable) birth defects must be aware of the complexity of causation and of the possible feelings of guilt and emotional trauma experienced by the parents involved (see Chapter 7 for information on counseling parents).

BRAIN DEVELOPMENT

In order to put environmental insult to cerebral development in perspective, a review of some recent important discoveries about brain development is necessary. The time of most rapid cell division and growth of a fetal organ is known as the *critical period*, and it is at this time that it is most vulnerable to insult (Wolff, 1970). The brain has a comparatively long critical period characterized by a complex series of specific critical periods for different sections of the developing brain. The nervous system is evident by 3 weeks, and the neural tube begins to close between 21 to 25 days. The most important period of neurological develop- ment is this first 10 weeks of intrauterine life when the anatomic, physiologic, and biochemical substrates of future development are being formed (Ferry, Culbertson, Fitzgibbons, & Netsky, 1979).

Because it is first to develop, the brain is disproportionate to the other body organs in early gestation, and within the brain, various sections grow at different rates. The medulla and pons, the largest region of the brain up to 7 weeks, become proportionately smaller at 18 weeks. The telencephalon is smaller than other regions at 4 weeks, but by 8 weeks it is growing more rapidly than any other part of the brain. The cerebellum has two spurts in growth, one at about 8 weeks of intrauterine life and the other in the 1st year after birth. The nerve fibers are protected by a cover of myelin, which transmits nerve impulses, essential for later cognitive interaction. The myelinization of nervous tissue begins in the 4th month of fetal life and is not complete until the 5th and 6th decades of postnatal life (Dodge, Prensky, & Feigin, 1975). With this pro- tracted developmental period, a prenatal insult that interrupts myelinization may not become apparent until later in childhood when the function of these myelinated pathways may be found to be defective (Ferry et al., 1979; Painter, 1979).

Hemispheric Specialization

Asymmetry of the brain is evident as early as 29 weeks gestation, which suggests that the substrate for language development in the left cerebral hemisphere is present well before birth (Ferry et al., 1979; Wada, Clarke, & Hamm, 1975). Hemispheric specialization continues throughout childhood with the right hemisphere specialized for nonsequential, spatial control and control of visual stimuli. The left hemisphere processes stimuli in a linguistic, se- quential, analytic manner to form the basis of receptive and ex- pressive language (Taylor, 1969; Witelson & Pallie, 1973). Dif- ferences are not absolute in that each side is able to execute some functions of the other. The brain's organization is less clear in left- handed people. The significance of hemispheric specialization for language learning has been pointed out by, among others, Pettit and Helms (1979) in research using dichotic listening. They found left hemispheric dominance for normal and articulation- disordered groups of children but no significant hemispheric dominance for a language-disordered group. This suggests that normal and articulation-disordered children have developed cerebral hemispheric dominance for language, while language disordered children may not have developed sufficient cerebral dominance for language learning. Given the specificity of the left hemisphere of the brain for language, it is reasonable that prenatal insult to the left temporal lobe may have potential, at least, for language problems. Causes of prenatal insult are discussed in the following sections.

NUTRITION AND FETAL GROWTH

Fetal malnutrition has been understood only recently, probably for two reasons, one technical and the other philosophical. The first was the relative inaccessibility of the fetus for observation. The second was the generally accepted view of the fetus as a perfect parasite, extracting what it needs from its mother and remaining unaffected by the mother's health, nutrition, or exposure to teratogens. Only a few years ago, obstetricians recommended strict weight control and even weight reduction in pregnancy. Recently, as researchers have begun to explore intrauterine conditions, these practices have been challenged (Stein & Susser, 1976; Winick, 1976).

An important biological principle was established by Winick and Noble (1966) in which they studied nutrition in rats. The critical period for brain development in rats is after birth. One group of rats was nutritionally deprived from birth to weaning; a second group was deprived for a similar period but after weaning. Both groups were then fed. The first group remained small with reduced head circumference while the second group caught up in weight to the weight of rats not deprived of nourishment. These results indicate that the *timing* of the malnutrition in development is critical to recovery from malnutrition.

Critical Period of Cell Division

Intrauterine environmental variables during the proliferative phase of cellular growth also have a part in determining the ultimate number of cells, not by altering the time during which cells can divide, but rather by altering the rate at which cell division occurs during the time prescribed by the genetic makeup of the animal. Malnutrition slows the rate of cell division, but cells do continue to divide for the same period of time in the malnourished animal as in the normal animal. Thus, the number of cells present in any organ at maturity is only partially under genetic control.

Malnutrition of the fetus at the time of most rapid increase in the number of cells may result in fewer cells. As in experimental animals, malnutrition may curtail cell division in any brain region undergoing formation. All brain cell types in the cerebrum, cerebellum, and brain stem so far studied are affected if they are dividing at the time the undernutrition occurs (Winick, 1976).

Critical Period of Cell Growth

Disruption of the formation of an organ during the critical period of formation clearly can be damaging. But even after the critical period of cell division has passed, the organ enters a significant growth phase in which it enlarges and the cells take on weight. The rate of weight gain is greater in the fetus between 26 and 36 weeks of gestation than at any other time in the human life span (Brooke, 1983). It is during this growth phase that nutrition plays a particularly important part. Enlargement of a fetal organ during the growing period results from an increase in the number of cells, an increase in the size of existing cells, or the simultaneous occurrence of both. Malnutrition at the time of growth in size of the individual cells may result in smaller cells, but those cells will expand to their normal size when they are properly nourished (Winick, 1976).

Effects of Low Birth Weight

If the fetus does not receive the needed nutrition, one obvious result is low birth weight. A newborn with low birth weight (LBW) is defined as weighing less than 1500g (5 lb). There are two reasons for LBW: the infant is premature and the right weight for its gestational age; or the infant is full term but is small for gestational age (SGA), either from primary or secondary growth deficiency. It has been recognized for several years that LBW is correlated with infant mortality and with high risk for developmental problems and neurodevelopmental abnormalities, which would include speech and language disorders (Drillien, 1964, 1967; Rubin, Rosenblatt, & Barlow, 1973; Stewart, Reynolds, & Lipscomb, 1981; Winsick, 1976). More recent studies suggest that developmental disorders are less frequent among LBW children than previously thought (Flower, 1981). The massive Collaborative Perinatal Project of the National Institute of Neurological and Communicative Disorders and Stroke (Vetter, Fay, & Winitz, 1980) showed significant differences in speech and language in only the very low-birth-weight infants.

Another obvious result of LBW is reduced head circumference. True microcephaly may be a result of fetal malnutrition or a sign of many other diseases and syndromes. Stein and Susser (1976) studied the effects of nutritional deprivation on the head circumferences of children delivered during the Dutch famine of 1944 to 1945. Head circumference was shown to be smaller in these prenatally malnourished children than in comparison groups.

Other studies indicate that head circumference is an important indicator of abnormal neurological and intellectual outcome. Gross, Kosmetatos, Grimes and Williams (1978) found mean IQ scores that were statistically lower together with a significantly higher rate of articulation defects for SGA children at age 4 who also had head circumferences between the 10th and 50th percentiles at birth. However, Martin (1970), in a large study of microcephalic babies, warned that the condition of microcephaly itself does not assure retardation. The incidence of normal intelligence in microcephalic children is not known, but it may be much higher than customarily thought.

Two studies separated the speech and language behavior of premature and SGA children for study. French, Marshall, and Sparks (1982) used a standardized test, the Sequenced Inventory of Communication Development, to compare premature, SGA, and normal children at 18 months. No significant differences were found between groups, but the number of subjects (10 per group) was small. Eaves, Nuttall, Klonoff, and Dunn (1970) compared 92 premature, 85 SGA, and 91 full-birth-weight children on the Griffiths Developmental Scale. They concluded that birth weight is the dominant factor determining the rate of mental development in LBW children in infancy, but socioeconomic status may become a more important factor later. There was no significant correlation between Griffiths scores at 6 months and Stanford-Binet scores at 4 years. As yet, it is not possible to predict from a test given in infancy which, if any, LBW children will have deficits in cognitive development.

Summary

Follow-up studies of speech and language in low-birth-weight infants are scarce. Results may be clouded by the effect that socioeconomic factors may have on the ability of the premature and SGA children's chances for catching up. The evidence does suggest that very low birth weight, whether in the premature or SGA child, is cause for concern about future cognitive development, and that future outcome is also at risk with reduced head circumference. Questions concerning birth weight, whether the child under 5 lb is full term or premature, are an important part of the case history. Given proper nutrition and stimulation, the premature infant would be expected to catch up, barring perinatal complications or injury, to developmental norms for speech and language. The child who is small for gestational age, however, may have a more serious problem. Causes of SGA are heterogeneous and include both primary and secondary growth failure.

Maternal Diabetes

There is a consensus that congenital anomalies are two to four times more frequent in the offspring of diabetic mothers than in those of nondiabetic women (Soler, Walsh, & Malins, 1976). Improvements in obstetric and neonatal care have enabled more infants of diabetic mothers (IDMs) to survive than was previously the case; and IDMs now represent nearly 1% of all live births on many obstetric services (Yogman, Cole, Als, & Lester, 1982). The anomalies of these infants do not appear to be specific, but commonly affected multiple organ systems (Bennett, Webner, & Miller, 1979).

The condition of diabetes itself, rather than genetic factors, appears to be the predominant determinant of the anomalies associated with diabetic pregnancies. The diabetic women most prone to have children with malformations are those who developed diabetes at an early age, have diabetes of long duration, are insulin treated, and have vascular complications (Bennett et al., 1979). Present evidence suggests that fetal anomalies are the result of metabolic disturbances in the uterine environment. For the duration of the pregnancy, the fetus is exposed to mild maternal hypoglycemia and hyperglycemia, which leads to continuous changes in fetal insulin output (Yogman et al., 1982). The above-average tendency for fetuses of diabetic mothers to be growth retarded between the 7th and 14th weeks of pregnancy (Pedersen, & Molsted-Pedersen, 1979) may account for the increased tendency of IDMs to have congenital malformations (Spiers, 1982).

Priestly (1972) studied the neurological status of newborn IDMs and found that they demonstrated decreased passive tone and increased tremulousness. Yogman et al., (1982) found that even those IDMs considered healthy by Day 3 behaved substantially differently on the Brazelton Neonatal Behavior Adjustment Scale than newborns of nondiabetic mothers. The IDMs showed poor head control while being pulled to sit, were tremulous, and readily changed skin color to a mottled or deep red. As social interactants, the IDMs had particular difficulty with visual orientation (attention to the human face alone and when combined with a voice). Their eye movements were jerky, and they had difficulty sustaining periods of alertness. The authors hypothesize that the behavior of the IDMs continues to be influenced postnatally by the exposure of their central nervous systems to high insulin levels in utero. They further hypothesize that the parents of these babies may have difficulties interacting with their non-visually-alert infants, particularly if parental anxieties have been heightened by a complicated pregnancy. Many of the parents described their babies as "difficult to get to know."

The intellectual development of IDMs from 8 months to 5 years has been studied by Churchill, Berendes, and Nemore (1969) as part of the Perinatal Collaborative Study and by Stehbens, Baker, and Kitchell (1977). Psychological evaluations were done using the Bayley Mental and Motor Scales and the Stanford Binet Intelligence Test. Both studies found IDMs to be more vulnerable to intellectual impairment, especially those infants who were born to acetone-positive diabetic mothers. The IDMs who were small for gestational age seemed particularly prone to long-term difficulty and had a higher incidence of congenital malformations. Unfortunately, data on language development were not reported separately in this study.

Clinicians should be concerned with maternal diabetes in a case history in that changes in infant behavior and responsiveness and intellectual impairment have been reported. At highest risk for intellectual impairment are IDMs who are also small for gestational age. Further research may identify IDMs as a group at high-risk for speech and language delay.

TERATOGENS

Teratogens are agents that produce or raise the incidence of congenital malformations (Thompson & Thompson, 1980). Only the offspring of the teratogen-exposed pregnancy will be affected. Not long ago, it was believed that the placenta served as a protective shield for the developing fetus. It is now known that nearly all substances taken by the mother during pregnancy are transferred across the placenta to the fetus. Nearly everything the mother consumes or breathes, the fetus consumes also.

However, not all fetuses exposed to a potential teratogen in utero will have birth defects, and the pattern of any abnormality as a consequence of a teratogen may vary. Some of the variation may result from exposure at different critical periods during gestation. Once the critical period for an organ has passed, the organ becomes insensitive to teratogens. For example, cleft palate cannot occur if exposure occurs after palatal closure.

Another important principle in the variation of the effect of teratogens is threshold. Threshold implies that a certain minimum amount of teratogen is required for a birth defect in a fetus. The thresholds for different mothers and fetuses will differ according to the health, nutrition, and genetics of the mother and the uterine environment and genetics of the fetus. There is a growing body of evidence suggesting that genetic makeup accounts for some of the differences in susceptibilities of fetuses to a teratogen (Phelan, Pellock, & Nance, 1982; Spielberg, 1982).

Some principles of teratology have been formulated by Pernoll, King, and Prescott (1980): (a) Susceptibility depends on the genotype of the fetus and the manner in which it interacts with environmental factors. Twins may differ in susceptibility to a teratogen. (b) Susceptibility to teratogenic agents varies with the developmental stage at the time of exposure (critical periods). (c) Teratogenic agents act in specific ways on developing cells. (d) The final manifestations of abnormal development due to teratogens are death, malformation, growth retardation, and functional disorders. (e) Manifestations of deviant development increase in degree as dosage increases from no-effect to totally lethal effect.

Radiation

The major physical agent that can cause birth defects is radiation. Radiation changes the chemical properties of the atoms and molecules within living cells and can cause birth defects in two ways: It can act as a mutagen to damage genes in sperm or egg cells so that genetic abnormalities may appear in later generations, or it can act as a teratogen to kill the cells of that particular developing embryo (Dooley, Russell, & Oldham, 1980; Shurtleff & Shurtleff, 1981).

The critical period for a fertilized egg to be killed by radiation is before it is implanted in the uterus. Either the embryo is destroyed or it develops normally. Radiation doses later, in the critical periods of organ formation, can cause malformations, growth retardation, and some embryo deaths. After this sensitive period has passed, higher concentrations are required to affect the phase of cell growth. Growth retardation is permanent and persists into adulthood. The later in pregnancy the radiation occurs, the greater the chance of catching up in growth (Barr, 1979; Strobino, Kline & Stein, 1978).

Besides the timing of the radiation dose at a particular stage of pregnancy, it is significant whether the total dose is received in a single burst, as several small doses, or continuously over an extended period (Dekaban, 1968). Divided doses and slow dose rates can greatly reduce the effects of a given total dose. Radiation that does not reach the unborn baby cannot directly affect it. If a pregnant woman undergoes skull X-rays, for example, and her abdomen is completely shielded, the procedure carries no known risk to the fetus.

It is generally believed that there is no threshold level below which radiation does no damage, although there are levels below which effects cannot be proved or measured. Some research suggests that at low doses, the mutational effect is less than expected (perhaps because cells' gene-repair mechanisms cope better with lesser amounts of damage) and that genetically damaged sperm and egg cells may be less likely to produce offspring (March of Dimes, 1979). An absorbed dose of 10 rads (radiation absorbed dose) by the fetus at any time during gestation is considered a practical threshold for the induction of congenital defects (Brent, 1976). The National Council of Radiation Protection and Measurement has recommended a maximal dose equivalent to 0.5 rad to the fetus from occupational exposure of pregnant women (Parker & Taylor, 1971). (See section on occupational hazards in this chapter.)

Prenatal radiation is a well-established cause of microcephaly and mental retardation (Dekaban, 1968; Miller & Blot, 1972). Children whose heads are deformed by radiation also have intrauterine growth retardation and, rarely, deformities of the extremities. Since the dangers have become recognized, radiation use during pregnancy is now rare, but there are still incidents of necessary radiation because of tumors in the mother.

There are no reports of specific speech and language behavior in children exposed to radiation prenatally. In the absence of data, significant prenatal radiation exposure in the case history should alert the clinician to the possibility of general growth retardation, which places a child in a high-risk category for signs of dysmorphology and developmental problems.

Alcohol: Fetal Alcohol Syndrome (FAS)

Alcohol has been a suspected teratogen for centuries, but only recently has a relationship been recognized between maternal alcohol intake and a characteristic pattern of malformation in the fetus: persisting growth deficiency of prenatal onset for length, weight, and brain; facial abnormalities, including epicanthic folds,

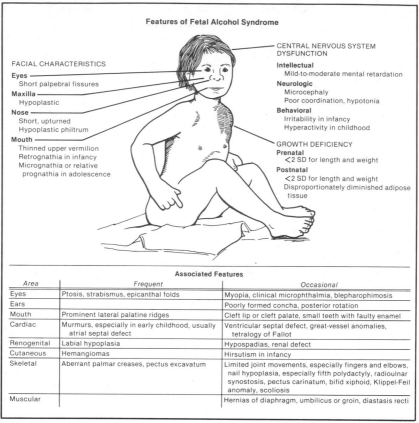

Features of Fetal Alcohol Syndrome

FACIAL CHARACTERISTICS

Eyes
Short palpebral fissures
Maxilla
Hypoplastic
Nose
Short, upturned
Hypoplastic philtrum
Mouth
Thinned upper vermilion
Retrognathia in infancy
Micrognathia or relative
prognathia in adolescence

CENTRAL NERVOUS SYSTEM
DYSFUNCTION
Intellectual
Mild-to-moderate mental retardation
Neurologic
Microcephaly
Poor coordination, hypotonia
Behavioral
Irritability in infancy
Hyperactivity in childhood

GROWTH DEFICIENCY
Prenatal
<2 SD for length and weight
Postnatal
<2 SD for length and weight
Disproportionately diminished adipose
tissue

Associated Features

Area	Frequent	Occasional
Eyes	Ptosis, strabismus, epicanthal folds	Myopia, clinical microphthalmia, blepharophimosis
Ears		Poorly formed concha, posterior rotation
Mouth	Prominent lateral palatine ridges	Cleft lip or cleft palate, small teeth with faulty enamel
Cardiac	Murmurs, especially in early childhood, usually atrial septal defect	Ventricular septal defect, great-vessel anomalies, tetralogy of Fallot
Renogenital	Labial hypoplasia	Hypospadias, renal defect
Cutaneous	Hemangiomas	Hirsutism in infancy
Skeletal	Aberrant palmar creases, pectus excavatum	Limited joint movements, especially fingers and elbows, nail hypoplasia, especially fifth polydactyly, radioulnar synostosis, pectus carinatum, bifid xiphoid, Klippel-Feil anomaly, scoliosis
Muscular		Hernias of diaphragm, umbilicus or groin, diastasis recti

FIGURE 5-1
From "The Fetal Alcohol Syndrome" by D.W. Smith, *Hospital Practice,*
Vol. 14, No. 10, October 1979. Illustration by Adele Spiegler.

thin upper lip, and small chin; delayed mental and motor development; and cardiac defects (JAMA, 1976; Streissguth, Herman &
Smith, 1978). Speech and language defects are often mentioned in
the medical literature, but there is little specific information as to
their nature. As Iosub, Fuchs, Bingol, Stone, and Gromisch (1981,
p.526) observe, "We have noted frequent speech and language abnormalities in children with FAS even in the absence of mental
retardation."

Diagnosis of FAS is especially difficult, because it is not an all-or-
none syndrome that can be identified prenatally or postnatally
with assurance. Affected children may not have any physical signs,
although those with most severe physical signs tend to have the

most severe mental handicaps. The clinician may be the first professional to suspect FAS if problems have not become apparent until the child enters school (Sparks, 1984).

The incidence of FAS has been estimated as 1 in 750 live births (Streissguth, Landesman-Dwyer, Martin, & Smith, 1980), making it one of the most common birth defects in the United States. The offspring of chronically alcoholic women are at highest risk, but clinical studies show that even moderate drinking during the first few weeks of pregnancy can adversely affect fetal development (Smith, 1979). Although FAS is clearly associated with chronic maternal alcoholism, the effects of individual drinking patterns, nutrition, smoking, drug use, genetic factors, metabolic differences, paternal alcoholism, and socioeconomic class are less well understood.

Exposure of the fetus to moderate or higher concentrations of alcohol is known to have differential effects at different stages of development. Alcohol, like other teratogens, appears to give rise to a spectrum of defects, and affected children may show great individual variation in both extent and severity of involvement. At one end of the spectrum are the more severely affected children in whom the basic diagnostic triad of growth deficiency, mental retardation, and facial abnormalities is fully exposed; yet equally important to the speech clinician as diagnostician are children with only partial or atypical expression of the syndrome. Perhaps the pertinent clinical question is not "Does this child have FAS?" but "Is this child's problem secondary to alcohol exposure in utero?" (Smith, 1979).

The intrauterine growth retardation in FAS is not completely understood. Because alcohol freely crosses the placenta, concentrations of alcohol in the fetus are at least as high as in the mother and probably have a toxic effect upon fetal organ development. Fisher et al. (1982) suggest that injury to the placenta induced by alcohol could lead to restriction of nutrients essential to fetal growth regardless of the state of maternal nutrition, that is, selective fetal malnutrition. Selectivity has been substantiated in studies of nonidentical twins by Christoffel and Salafsky (1975) and identical twins by Palmer, Ouellette, Warner, and Leichtman (1974). Discordance of anomalies was found in both studies, leading to speculation by the authors that the fetuses had different susceptabilities to the influence of alcohol in utero, and, therefore, a direct cause and effect between amount of alcohol ingested and the severity of the features of FAS cannot be drawn.

The major impact of alcohol is growth deficiency resulting from a diminished number of cells. The growth deficiency is disharmonic; it is more striking in brain and eye development than in linear growth and more pronounced in midfacial growth than in general skeletal growth. The infants are born small for gestational age with a head size that is even further reduced in relation to their reduced length. Contrary to what might be expected, however, they are usually not underweight for their length at birth. Characteristically, in the FAS baby the eyes are undersized, and the palpebral fissures (eyeslits) are comparatively short. The midface is small, giving a relatively flat lateral facial contour, and there is an indistinct philtrum (the ridges running between the nose and the lips).

Postnatally, these infants continue to grow at a slow pace and tend to become underweight for their length. The rate of linear growth is about two thirds the normal rate, and weight gain may drop to half the normal rate. Such infants are often hospitalized for evaluation of nutrition, but hospitalization, foster care, or good home care does not produce improvement. This failure to catch up to normal growth rates is a consistent diagnostic feature (Smith, 1979).

Mental retardation of varying degrees is the most debilitating characteristic of FAS. Several authors state that the impact on brain dysfunction in FAS is directly related to the severity of the physical features; the most severely affected children also have the greatest intellectual handicap (Iosub et al., 1981; Jones, Smith, Streissguth, & Myrianthopoulos, 1974; Streissguth et al., 1978).

Streissguth et al. (1978) reported psychological measurements on 20 cases, ages 9 months to 21 years, with severe to very mild physical signs of FAS and varied socioeconomic class and postnatal care. Their testing is of special interest to speech-language pathologists because of the language emphasis in the tests used: the Bayley Scale of Infant Development, the Stanford-Binet, and the Wechsler Intelligence Scale. The subjects were found to range from normal intelligence to severe mental retardation with a mean IQ level of 65. The IQ scores of the children were inversely related to the severity of their physical evidence of FAS: The most severely affected children had the lowest average IQ (55); the moderately affected group averaged 58 IQ; and the group diagnosed as having mild FAS had the highest average IQ scores (82). The three children in the normal range had personality and adjustment problems that interfered with success in school.

On the other hand, some investigators have reported cognitive or intellectual deficits in children born to alcoholic mothers but lacking physical characteristics of FAS (Olegard, Sabel, & Aronsson 1979; Jones et al., 1974). Clarren and Smith (1978) reported autopsies of the offspring of four alcoholic and "binge" drinking mothers and reported that two showed no external FAS characteristics while all four had similar brain malformations stemming from errors in migration of neuronal and glial elements. Clarren and Smith concluded that in some infants problems of brain structure and/or function may occur as the only apparent abnormality in the wake of intrauterine alcohol exposure.

The child with FAS is subject to central nervous system disorders, such as delayed motor development, tremulousness, and perceptural-motor disturbances. He or she is likely to need special education services, including speech and language therapy, for the related behavior problems of hyperactivity and poor attention span. Streissguth et al. (1980) described the behavior of many of their sample of 20 children as hyperactive in their preschool years. Those with less hyperactivity were distractible and had short attention spans. Hyperactivity appears to be one of those symptoms that may or may not appear in FAS children. Aside from hyperactivity, none of the 20 children was reported to have serious behavior problems of an antisocial or psychotic nature. Two of the children who appeared to be very withdrawn and fearful became hyperactive when removed from their alcoholic mothers and placed in a more nurturing environment. School problems stemming from both learning difficulties and hyperactivity were frequent in this sample group, even in one subject with normal intelligence.

Signs of central nervous system disorders are also evident in the behavior of newborn FAS children, including hyperacusis (heightened sensitivity to sound), irritability (which may result from withdrawl from alcohol), atypical head orientation, and decreased body activity. Weak sucking ability and other feeding difficulties are common in the 1st year of life (Pierog, Chandavasu, & Wexler, 1977).

The only descriptions of speech and language in FAS children are the observation of medical investigators. Iosub et al., (1981) report some observations in their study of three children in one family. All three children were born to a woman who began to drink 1 1/2 qt of whiskey per day while a teenager, before the birth of her first child, and continued through the birth of her third child at age 31. The three children exhibited the cardinal features of FAS: growth deficiency, microcephaly, mental retardation, facial characteristics, and hyperactivity. Two of the children had malocclusion and micronathia. The descriptions of the speech of these two were "monotonous voice, speech slightly slurred" for one and "she has speech and language abnormalities, consisting of voice dysfunction, disorders of articulation, and fluency problems" for the other (p.525). The third child had a cleft palate.

Streissguth et al. (1978) reported one subject, a classroom management problem, with "loose associations and unintelligible verbalizations intermingled with appropriate speech" (p.365).

Several authors reported no change in physical or mental symptoms despite changes for the better in the care and stimulation the FAS children received. Hanson, Jones, & Smith (1976) report that in 41 cases studied, there was no indication of catch-up growth or performance during infancy and early childhood. Affected babies who had been raised in foster care and received multiple services from early infancy had shown no better growth or performance in general than those raised by the chronically alcoholic mother. A long-term—follow-up study (Iosub et al., 1981) emphasizes the lack of catch-up growth even with adequate nutrition and emotional stimulation. Repeated IQ tests over a 10 year period showed that their three patients' mental states and IQs remained largely the same regardless of environmental changes for the better.

Of prognostic interest also are two of the subjects from the study by Streissguth et al. (1978). Both were young men, 20 and 21 years old, friendly, and outgoing. Adult heights and head circumferences were 2 standard deviations below the mean; both were retarded and required sheltered environments. One of them (IQ 67) from a welfare background had been institutionalized for most of his life. The other (IQ 57) was born to well-educated professionals and raised by his own loving and affluent family. In these two adults, neither mental nor physical catch-up growth occurred.

This inability to catch up either mentally or physically can be contrasted with studies of children who have prenatal malnutrition syndrome without alcohol (McKay, Sinisterra, McKay, Gomez, & Lloreda, 1978; Winick, 1976). These children were also born severely underweight, but when given proper nutrition and mental stimulation, they did catch up physically and mentally to infants of normal birth weight.

Summary

In view of the suspected high incidence of FAS, the lack of data concerning its effect on speech and language development handicaps clinicians in therapy. FAS can occur in the absence of physical signs, but those children with the most severe signs are those most severely affected mentally. Growth deficiency and a characteristic face are cardinal diagnostic signs. It is not known if language development is consistent with overall developmental delay or has another characteristic pattern. Prognosis is poor for improvement in cognition even when the child receives good care and intellectual stimulation.

Drugs as Teratogens

A few drugs have been proved positively to cause predictable birth defects while others are only suspected. Few are as obvious as the epidemic in .1961 of limb-reduction malformations in newborns due to maternal ingestion early in pregnancy of the sedative thalidomide. This finding had obstetric, legal, pharmaceutical, and governmental regulatory repercussions that are still continuing.

It is difficult to assign specific cause to specific drugs for several reasons: (a) The drug may be administered as therapy for an illness that itself causes the malformation. (b) The fetal malformation may cause maternal symptoms that are treated with a specific drug. (c) The drug may inhibit the abortion of an already-malformed infant. (d) The drug may commonly be employed in combination with a second drug, which causes a malformation (Golbus, 1980). In the summaries of teratogenic drugs that follow, their effects on speech and language are not included, because information is not available. The discussion of the drugs is intended as a resource for the clinician who finds prenatal drug history in a patient.

Antithyroid agents

The most common result of hypothyroidism in the infant is congenital cretinism, associated with mental retardation and found in children of chronically hypothyroid mothers and in cases of maternal therapy with antithyroid compounds. Cretinism can be mistaken for Down syndrome by its phenotype. Like Down syndrome, it can be detected by amniocentesis, although there is no chromosomal abnormality associated with it. Unlike Down syndrome, it can be successfully treated in infancy and mental retardation avoided with early detection (Golbus, 1980).

Anticonvulsants and fetal hydantoin syndrome

The National Institutes of Health (From the NIH, 1981) estimate that approximately 1 per 200 pregnant women is epileptic, and anticonvulsant drug therapy is usually continued throughout pregnancy. Exposure of the fetus to anticonvulsants introduces a twofold to fivefold increase in the risk of having an infant with anomalies, with specific increases in oral clefts and congenital heart defects. Of the more than 16 drugs on the market for seizures, phenobarbital is safest for the fetus and is the drug of choice for pregnant women with epilepsy (Golbus, 1980).

Dilantin and closely related compounds (hydantoins) used to control seizures are potentially harmful to the fetus. The manifestations of fetal hydantoin syndrome are similar to those of fetal alcohol syndrome. As in FAS, mental retardation is the most debilitating manifestation. Smith (1982) reports that infants with fetal hydantoin syndrome who show multiple hydantoin effects have an average IQ of 71. It should be noted, however, that unlike FAS, mental performance in childhood may improve after poor performance early in infancy. Other manifestations are: mild-to-moderate growth deficiency, usually of prenatal onset, coupled with failure to thrive in the early postnatal months; characteristic facial features, including low and broad nasal bridge; widely spaced eyes; coarse hair; and small or missing nails on both feet and hands (Smith, 1982).

The risk of the exposed fetus having fetal hydantoin syndrome is about 10%, and the risk for having some effects of the disorder is an additional 33 percent. No dose-response curve has been demonstrated, nor has a "safe" dose been found below which there is no teratogenic risk.

Cancer therapy drugs

Drugs for the treatment of cancer, especially aminopterin, have been linked to fetal malformations (Schafer, 1981). These agents work best against rapidly dividing cells and are effective not only against cancerous growth but against the developing fetus as well. Golbus (1980) identified these compounds among the most potent teratogens known.

Cigarette Smoking

Though not a teratogen in the usual sense of producing malformations, it is now widely recognized that maternal smoking in pregnancy is associated with both reduction in birth weight and increased perinatal mortality. In addition, there is evidence that the decreased birth weight of offspring of smokers is independent of race, parity (number of previous children), age, and socioeconomic status, and is directly proportional to the number of cigarettes smoked (dose-response curve). The effect disappears in subsequent pregnancies if the mother does not smoke (Rush, 1974; Simpson, 1957).

Two components of smoke, nicotine and carbon monoxide, are the agents most likely to affect fetal growth. Nicotine has been linked to decreased uterine blood flow and decreased fetal breathing movements. Carbon monoxide crosses the placenta to reduce fetal oxygen. The combination of acute uterine vasoconstriction (nicotine induced) and a decrease in fetal oxygen supply (carbon monoxide induced) are likely to be additive (ACOG, 1979).

There is no reported evidence of specific speech and language difficulty in children tied directly to maternal smoking during pregnancy, but there is some suggestion that fetal central nervous system development, as well as growth pattern, may be impaired as a result of maternal smoking. Butler and Goldstein (1973) reported a height deficit of 1 cm at the ages of 7 and 11 in children whose mothers smoked 10 or more cigarettes per day after the 4th month of pregnancy, and a 3- to 5- month delay in reading, mathematics and general ability after allowing for associated social and biological factors.

Social Drugs

Two large studies (Golbus, 1980; Vorhees, Brunner, & Butcher, 1979) have demonstrated that there is no increased risk of congenital anomalies per se from narcotic addiction of the mother, but the neonates have high incidence of intrauterine growth retardation and breech delivery, while their mothers experience increased incidence of such perinatal complications as toxemia and premature labor.

Wilson, McCreary, Kean, & Baxter (1979) studied 3- to 6-year-old children of heroin-addicted mothers and found that they did not differ significantly on the verbal or motor scales of the McCarthy Scales of Children's Abilities or on the receptive or expressive measures of the Illinois Test of Psycholinguistic Abilities from normal children. However, the heroin-exposed children scored significantly lower on the subtests measuring organization on both tests. Behaviorally, these children had problems of impulsiveness, aggressiveness, and poor peer relations. The authors concluded that chronic uterine exposure to heroin may affect perceptual and learning processes as well as growth and behavior in preschool children. It appears that more behavioral problems would be expected in these children than speech and language problems.

LSD has been reviewed extensively (Dumas, 1971; Golbus, 1980; Jacobson & Berlin, 1972). Mothers who use LSD have a history of multiple-drug ingestion, poor nutrition in the 1st trimester of pregnancy, and cigarette smoking, and they are generally a high-risk group for perinatal complications. There is evidence of chromosomal breakage in newborns of mothers who use LSD, but it is contradictory. Jacobson and Berlin found breakage in 50% of the newborns of LSD-using parents, but the breakage was repaired in their chromosomes by 3 to 6 months. Dumas examined the chromosomes of a comparable group and found no breakage. Jacobson and Berlin also found an incidence of major congenital anomalies, chiefly in the central nervous system, in 96 per 1,000 live births of LSD using parents, or 10 to 20 times that expected for the American population. However, the authors note these defects may be multifactorial in nature. Prenatal environmental factors, especially infections, may account for as much of the high risk of this group as alterations in the DNA as a result of LSD acting as a teratogen or mutagen.

There is no evidence that marijuana is a human teratogen but there is also no assurance that marijuana exposure is safe for the fetus (Golbus, 1980).

INFECTIONS

Bacterial infections that attack the mother, the placenta, and the fetus, such as syphilis and gonorrhea, were essentially eliminated with the advent of antibiotics. However, some resistant strains have appeared and are increasing rapidly again (Shurtleff & Shurtleff, 1981). Syphilis interferes with embryonic development and causes destruction of already formed organs. Gonorrhea is most commonly transmitted to the neonate at the time of delivery and does not cause the type of birth defects that involve speech and language.

There are a few viruses that warrant special attention. Herpes Type 2 (venereal) can cause intrauterine disease late in pregnancy or be transmitted to the baby at birth (Brent, 1976), although cesarean section delivery avoids infecting the neonate. Fetal and infant infections of herpes Type 2 are associated with severe destruction of the nervous system (Shurtleff & Shurtleff, 1981). The cytomegalovirus is common, but it rarely affects the fetus or newborn. It is capable of producing encephalitis and malformations of the brain (Shurtleff & Shurtleff, 1981).

Congenital Rubella Syndrome

Because of the extent of the devastation of the fetus by maternal rubella infection, this virus warrants special attention. Immunization for rubella was introduced in 1969, but the children born during the rubella outbreak of 1963 to 1965 are still receiving attention from clinicians. Congenital rubella is a chronic contagious viral disease that begins in fetal life and continues into childhood for an unknown period. Hearing impairment is the most common manifestation and may be progressive, but disorders of the heart, eyes, and brain (retardation and developmental disability) are also common. The virus is widely disseminated within the tissues of the fetus and resides in the cell nucleus. The main mechanisms for production of malformation are cell death or a decreased rate of cell growth, or both. Rubella is variable in manifestation depending on the critical period in which it is contracted. The potential for defect is highest if the virus infects the fetus during the first 3 months. The damage to the child following rubella contracted in the 2nd trimester may not be as obvious in the newborn period (Cherry, 1980; Desmond, 1967).

Besides the obvious problems of rubella syndrome, Desmond (1967) reports more subtle manifestations of the disorder that are also characteristic of brain-damaged children: hyperactivity, impulsivity, poor attention span, sleep disturbances, delayed acquisition of living skills, and poor language development.

OCCUPATIONAL HAZARDS

An increasing proportion of women continue to work during pregnancy, and this trend seems likely to continue. Therefore, attention must be given by clinicians to external environmental hazards that are thought to affect the fetus in certain occupations.

In occupations involving X-rays, such as medical radiology, checking metal equipment in industry, or examining baggage in airports, the protective screening provided may not be adequate and thus may allow some fetal exposure (Chamberlain, 1981). Pregnant women are excluded from working in operating rooms because of the increased incidence of spontaneous abortion and

TABLE 5-1
Hazardous substances affecting reproductive function. From *Occupational Medicine: Surveillance, Diagnosis and Treatment.* by M.H. Turk, (Ed.), F. and S. Press, A division of Frost and Sullivan, Inc., 1982. Reprinted by permission.

Hazardous substances affecting reproductive function

Substance	Suspected Effects	Exposure Limits
Benzene	Teratogen	Minimal during pregnancy
Carbaryl	Teratogen	Minimal during pregnancy
Carbon disulfide	Teratogen	Minimal during pregnancy
Carbon tetrachloride	Teratogen	Minimal during pregnancy
Chloroform	Teratogen	Minimal during pregnancy
Chloroprene	Teratogen	Minimal during pregnancy
DBCP	Sterility	
Dioxin		
Endrin	Congenital defects	Minimal during pregnancy
Ethylene dibromide	Mutagen	
Ethylene dichloride	Toxic	Minimal during lactation
Ethylene oxide	Sterility/mutagenicity	Male
Ethylene thiourea	Mutagen/teratogen	Minimal during pregancy
Glycidyl ethers	Mutagen	
Herbicides, general		
Hexachlorophene	Suspected teratogen	Minimal during pregnancy
Lead	Birth defects	Minimal in females of child-bearing age
Mercury		
Pesticides, general		
Polychlorinated biphenyls	Toxic	Minimal during lactation
Tetrachloroethylene	Congenital abnormalities	Minimal during pregnancy
Waste anesthetic gases and vapors		Minimal during pregnancy

congenital anomalies in the offspring of operating room personnel (Cohen et al., 1974; Spense, Cohen, & Brown, 1977). Those occupations that expose pregnant women to low concentrations of various compounds over a long term also pose a threat to the developing fetus; lead and mercury are established teratogens resulting in various malformations, growth retardation, cerebral palsy, and microcephaly. Cadmium, nickel and selenium are heavy metals that have also been implicated as teratogens (Longo, 1980). (See Table 5-1)

POLLUTANTS

Pollution and contamination of the air, food, and water are the result of technological progress in an advancing society. America synthesizes tens of thousands of new chemicals each year (Ajl, 1982), and most of those are soon found on farms and in food and water supplies. The problems that result may be solved through further technology, which, in turn, will bring more teratogens and mutagens into the environment, which will require further solutions in an endless cycle (Golbus, 1980). The questions raised about the rights of the fetus and the rights and responsibilities of women, industry, and the state, grow ever more complex and will not be addressed here, but they will be of increasing concern to all health professionals, including those who work with communication problems.

Case History When a Teratogen is Suspected

When a teratogen is suspected as the cause of a child's condition, the usual perfunctory history will probably not uncover any useful information. Let us use alcohol consumption and suspected fetal alcohol syndrome as an example. If the child is within normal limits on the height/weight/head circumference charts, the pediatrician may be unaware of any problems until the child has difficulty with speech and language or with school. Even careful history taking by the clinician may yield no information other than that the birth was uneventful, the pregnancy was normal, and the child has been in good health since. Reluctance to question in this area is pervasive in health professionals who might be considered sophisticated with alcoholic patients. Clinicians are often reluctant to offend the patient by searching for evidence of alcohol abuse. The mother's denial, not only to others but to herself, results in considerable resistance to providing information. This denial is part of any alcohol problem and therefore should be considered a symptom.

Clinicians may profit from the following guidelines to avoid resistance when taking the history (Sokol, Miller, & Martier, 1982). If the history taking process begins with, or is limited to, finding out the volume of alcohol consumed by the mother, it is unlikely that the clinician will elicit useful information. Failure is assured if the clinician asks "You didn't drink, did you?" What is communicated is the clinician's desire to avoid the issue. Because of the guilt, denial, and stigma the mother may already feel, the "How much did you drink?" approach can result in increased resistance to providing any data at all. This approach is not recommended.

A nonjudgmental, accepting, and concerned attitude is para-mount in gaining cooperation and, thus, in taking the family history. Along with questions about diabetes, genetic history, and speech or hearing problems, the clinician can ask, "Has anybody in your family had a drinking problem?" This paves the way for further indirect inquiry. The clinician then focuses questioning on the prepregnancy history of the mother.

The question "When did you first start drinking?" may bring an answer that drinking began in the early teenage years. The natural lead is then: "How much did you drink at that time?" "Did you ever get into trouble because of drinking?" and "How much could you hold at that time?" Rather than ask "How much did you drink when you were pregnant?", ask "How much could you drink at one time?" or "How much could you hold at that time?" Women who abuse alcohol will often report that they can consume, without getting drunk, what the light-to-moderate drinker might consider to be truly prodigious amounts of alcohol.

To obtain an accurate assessment, it is often helpful to suggest a range of expected responses to the woman. The key here is to sug-gest relatively high amounts. The communication to the mother is that it is alright to tell how much she drinks; it is a routine disclosure. Obviously, questioning to this point will not be war-ranted if it seems by the answers that the woman is not an alcohol abuser. As in other parts of history taking, positive responses should lead to further questions. With increasing experience, the process of taking a history of alcohol abuse becomes more efficient.

The case history format for suspected ingestion of socially used drugs should follow the same pattern. Disclosure by the mother of the nonelective ingestion of teratogens is not likely to elicit the defenses that are present in the alcoholic or drug-using mother. Appropriate referrals for counseling may be made for the parents who have questions and/or need to deal with unaccustomed or long-buried feelings of guilt. An evaluation format provided in the Appendices is recommended for the child with an environmental birth defect.

Case Report

Susan was referred to the WMU Language Speech and Hearing Clinic by her pediatrician at the age of 21 months because she had a very short attention span and did not talk or seem to comprehend speech. At birth Susan weighed 8 lb 10 oz and had a minor heart murmur. Though Susan had normal pure tone hearing, she seemed unable to comprehend any commands such as "Come here" or "Stand still." Her parents reported that she looked as if she did not understand what was being said. At age 2, her language skills were judged to be at about 12 months, with a severe receptive deficit.

At 26 months of age, Susan received an occupational therapy evaluation. A general developmental level could not be determined as the levels of all behaviors were diverse with exceptions to each level of testing. Her best score was her gross motor score of 21 months on the Gesell Developmental Schedule. All other scores on the Gesell and the Denver Developmental Screening Test ranged from 13 to 18 months. A possible diagnosis of infantile autism was suggested to her parents by her pediatrician.

At age 4, Susan was given a neurological evaluation at a large university hospital. She was noted to be clumsy, she knocked things over because she misjudged distances, and she had difficulty walking up steps. Her record from that evaluation noted that she was lethargic, reserved and independent and did not like to be held as a baby. She was noted to have said a few words when she was 20 months of age but did not begin persistent babbling until she was 2-3 years old and was receiving speech therapy. The neurological evaluation, computerized tomography (CT) brain scan and electroencephalogram (EEG) showed no pathology. The diagnosis was developmental aphasia.

Susan received speech and language therapy concurrently with occupational therapy from ages 2 to 4 when she was placed in a day-long program of total special education at a school that included those services. Throughout the next several years of puzzling episodes with Susan, the question of etiology arose again and again, both from her parents and from her clinicians. In all records from physicians (neurologist, pediatricians) as well as from psychologists and special educators, the birth history was recorded as "normal" and the mother's health as "excellent" during pregnancy. Although her mother was obviously obese, this fact was not mentioned in Susan's records. It was not until several years later that Susan's mother was comfortable about discussing the pregnancy with a clinician. Before she became pregnant she had taken LSD as a "social drug" a total of 14 times. She became pregnant with her first child who was normal and has been free of problems. Susan was the second of three children. The mother described that pregnancy as being the "worst time of my life." She suffered from compulsive overeating. She ate 3 to 4 lb of sugar each day, usually in the form of chocolates. Consumption of this amount of sugar may have depleted her body of the vitamins and minerals necessary for nutrition of the fetus. In addition, she stated that she had smoked one pack of cigarettes per day and had 10 alcoholic binges during her pregnancy. Contrary to an "excellent" prenatal history, there are a number of reasons to suspect interference with normal brain development: malnutrition, alcohol abuse, heavy smoking, and LSD use. Apparently no one had asked. Even so, it must be noted that there is no clear-cut cause-and-effect relationship on Susan from the many suspected environmental interferences with her prenatal development.

Therapy with Susan was a frustrating experience for both the clinician and the patient. A consistent reinforcer could not be found. Susan had days when she seemed unreachable; a goal that had been accomplished seemed forgotten, and she stared blankly at the clinician. The fact that Susan looked so healthy and normal only increased the clinician's bewilderment. A combination of highly structured operant therapy for half the session, followed by a play therapy period for communicative interaction, proved most effective. The structured part was based on Eisenson's treatment of aphasia in children (Eisenson, 1972) by building concepts of representational behavior in careful steps from matching like objects, to matching pictures, to categorizing functions. Therapy for expressive vocabulary was based on naming the objects and functions. An example is a therapy session at age 4 1/2:
Objective: Expressive vocabulary.

1. Susan, given action pictures, will correctly name the action when asked by the clinician "What is the boy/girl/children or family doing?" in 3/5 trials.

2. Susan, given familiar objects, will name their function: "What do you do with the soap? With the pencil? With the comb?" in 3/5 trials.

3. Susan will verbalize during play therapy. The clinician will engage in solo play with dolls and other toys. Susan will join in, asking for the objects she wants to play with and verbalizing what she is doing with baby or the toys.

At age 7 Susan had still another diagnosis, trainable mentally impaired, and was in a public school special education program. Her receptive language was estimated to be at the 5-year level. She was able to respond to three-part commands if she was given time to process slowly. She could count to 15, recognize numbers and letters, and write her name with prompting. Her performance was reported as uneven with some skills at the 4-year level and others at the 7-year level.

Summary

Susan's case illustrates three important implications for clinicians: (a) the difficulty in obtaining an accurate case history, (b) the reluctance of all health professionals to ask pertinent questions, and (c) the complexity of etiology. The lack of a definitive diagnosis was, and remains, the major problem. Even though a cause-and-effect relationship between prenatal history and the disorder may not be clear, her prenatal history cannot contribute in any way to diagnosis, therapy, or prognosis if it is not known.

REFERENCES

ACOG. Cigarette smoking and pregnancy. *American College of Obstetricians and Gynecologists Technical Bulletin,* 1979, *53,* 1-4.

Ajl, S.J. Birth defects research: 1980 and after. *American Journal of Medicine,* 1982, *72,* 119-126.

Barr, M. *Radiation hazards and the unborn.* Paper presented at the March of Dimes Conference on Birth Defects, Detroit, October, 1979.

Bennett, P.H., Webner, C., & Miller, M. Congenital anomalies and the diabetic and prediabetic pregnancy. Pregnancy, metabolism, diabetes and the fetus. *Excerpta Medica.* Amsterdam: Ciba Foundation symposium, 1979.

Brent, R.L.: Environmental factors. Radiation. In R.L. Brent & M.I. Harris (Eds.), *Prevention of embryonic, fetal and perinatal disease, Fogarty International Center Series on Preventive Medicine, (DHEW Publication No ((NIH)) 76-853), Bethesda, MD,* 1976, 3, 179-197.

Brooke, O.G. Nutrition in the pre-term infant. *Lancet,* 1983, *1,* 514-515.

Butler, N.R., & Goldstein, H. Smoking in pregnancy and subsequent child development. *British Medical Journal,* 1973, *4,* 573-575.

Chamberlain, G. Pregnant women at work, *Lancet,* 1983, *1,* 228-230.

Cherry, J.D. The new epidemiology of measles and rubella. *Hospital Practice,* 1980, 15:7, 49-57.

Christoffel, K.K., & Salafsky, I. Fetal alcohol syndrome in dizygotic twins. *Pediatrics,* 1975, *87,* 963-967.

120   *Birth Defects and Speech-Language Disorders*

Churchill, J.A., Berendes, H.W., & Nemore, J. Neuropsychological deficits in children of diabetic mothers. *American Journal of Obstetrics and Gynecology*, 1969, *145*, 247-268.

Clarren, S.K., & Smith, D.W. The fetal alcohol syndrome. *The New England Journal of Medicine*, *298*, 1978, 1063-1067.

Cohen, E.N., Brown, B.W., Jr., Bruce, D.L., Cascorbi, H.F., Corbett, T.H., Jones, T.W., & Whitcher, C.E. Occupational disease among 3 operating room personnel: A national study. *Anesthesiology*, 1974, *35*, 343.

Dekaban, A.S. Abnormalities in children exposed to x-radiation during various stages of gestation: Tentative timetable of radiation injury to the human fetus. *Journal of Nuclear Medicine*, 1968, 9 (Suppl. 1), 471-477.

Desmond, M.M. Congenital rubella encephalitis. *Journal of pediatrics*, 1967, *71*, 311-331.

Dodge, P.R., Prensky, A.L. & Feigin, R.D. Morphologic development. In P.R. Dodge, A.L. Prensky & R.D. Feigin (Eds.), *Nutrition and the developing nervous system* (Chapter 1) St. Louis: Mosby, 1975.

Dooley, W.C., Russell, M.H. & Oldham, R.K. Possible association between radiation exposure and chromosome changes. *Lancet*, 1980, (2),98.

Drillien, C.M. *The growth and development of the prematurely born infant.* Edinburgh, Scotland: Livingstone, 1964.

Drillien, C.M. The incidence of mental and physical handicaps in school age children of very low birth weight. *Pediatrics*, 1967, *39*, 238-247.

Dumas, K.W., Jr. Parental drug usage: Effect upon chromosomes of progeny. *Pediatrics*, 1971, 47:1037.

Eaves, L.C., Nuttall, J.C., Klonoff, H., & Dunn, H.G. Developmental and psychological test scores in children of low birth weight. *Pediatrics*, 1970, *45*(1), 9-20.

Eisenson, J. *Aphasia in children.* New York: Harper & Row, 1972.

Ferry, P.C., Culbertson, J.L., Fitzgibbons, P.M., & Netsky, M.G. Brain function and language disabilities. *International Journal of Pediatric Otorhinolaryngology*, 1979, *1*, 13-24.

Fisher, S.E., Atkinson, M., Burnap, J.K., Jacobson, S., Sehgal, P.K., Scott, ,W., & Van Thiel, D.H. Ethanol-associated selective fetal malnutrition: A contributing factor in the fetal alcohol syndrome. *Alcoholism: Clinical and Experimental Research*, 1982, *6*(2), 197-201.

Flower, R.M. Neurodevelopmental disorders in children. In J.K. Darby, Jr. (Ed.) *Speech evaluation in medicine.* New York: Grune & Stratton, 1981.

French, C., Marshall, L. & Sparks, S. Pre-linguistic differences of premature and small for gestational age infants. Paper presented to the American Speech-Language Hearing Association, Toronto, November, 1982.

From the NIH. Anticonvulsants found to have teratogenic potential. *Journal of the American Medical Association*, 1981, *245*(1), 36.

Golbus, M.S. Teratology for the obstetrician: Current status. *Obstetrics and Gynecology*, 1980, *55*(3), 1-9.

Gross, S.J., Kosmetatos, N., Grimes, C.T., & Williams, M.L. Newborn head size and neurological status: Predictors of growth and development of low birth weight infants. *Americn Journal of Diseases of Children*, 1978, *132*, 753-756.

Hanson, J.W., Jones, K.L., & Smith, D.W. Fetal alcohol syndrome, experience with 44 patients. *Journal of American Medical Association*, 1976, *235*, 1458-1460.

Iosub, ,S., Fuchs, M., Bingol, N., Stone, R.K., & Gromisch, D.S. Long term follow-up of three siblings with fetal alcohol syndrome. *Alcoholism: Clinical and Experimental Research*, 1981, *5*(4), 523-527.

Jacobson, C.B. & Berlin, C.M. Possible reproductive detriment in LSD users. *Journal of the American Medical Association*, 1972, *222*, 1367-1373.

JAMA Medical News. Heart defects accompany fetal alcohol syndrome. *Journal of the American Medical Association*, 1976, *235*, 2073.

Jones, K.L., Smith, D.W., Streissguth, A.P., & Myrianthopoulos, N.C. Outcome in offspring of chronic alcoholic women. *Lancet*, 1974, *1*, 1076-1078.

Longo, L.D. Environmental pollution and pregnancy: Risks and uncertainties for the fetus and infant. *American Journal of Obstetrics and Gynecology*, 1980, *137*(2), 162-173.

March of Dimes Science News Information File. *Radiation and birth defects*. White Plains, NY: March of Dimes, 1979.

Martin, H.P. Microcephaly and mental retardation. *American Journal of Diseases of Children*, 1970, *119*, 128.

McKay, H., Sinisterra, L., McKay, A., Gomez, H., & Lloreda, P. Improving cognitive ability in chronically deprived children. *Science*, 1978, *200*(21), 270-278.

Miller, R.W. & Blot, W.J. Small head size following in-utero exposure to atomic radiation. *Lancet*, 1972, *2*, 784-787.

Olegard, R., Sabel, K.G., & Aronsson, M. Effects on the child of alcohol abuse during pregnancy. Retrospective and prospective studies. *Acta Paediatrica Scandinavica*, 1979, *275*, 112-121.

Painter, M.J. Neurologic sequalae of birth. In J.J. Sciarria (Ed.), *Gynecology and Obstetrics: Vol. 3* (Chapter 99). Hagerstown, MD: Harper & Row, 1979.

Palmer, R.H., Ouellette, E.M., Warner, L., & Leichtman, S.R. Congenital malformations in offspring of a chronically alcoholic mother. *Pediatrics*, 1974, *53*, 490.

Parker, H.M. & Taylor, L.S. *Basic radiation protection criteria* Report No. 39, 1971. Washington, DC: National Council on Radiation Protection and Measurements.

Pedersen, J., & Molsted-Pedersen, I. Congenital malformations: The possible role of diabetes care outside pregnancy. In Pregnancy metabolism, diabetes and the fetus. (Ciba Foundation Symposium 63). *Excerpta Medica*. Amsterdam: Ciba Foundation symposium, 1979.

Pernoll, M.L., King, C.R., & Prescott, G.H. Genetics for the clinical obstetrician-gynecologist. *Obstetrics and Gynecology Annual*, 1980, *9*, 1-53.

Pettit, J.M., & Helms, S.B. Hemispheric language dominance of language-disordered, articulation-disordered, and normal children. *Journal of Learning Disabilities*, 1979, *12*, 12-17.

Phelan, M.C., Pellock, M.M., & Nance, W.E. Discordant expression of fetal hydantoin syndrome in heteropaternal dizygotic twins. *New England Journal of Medicine*, 1982, *307*(2), 99-101.

Pierog, S., Chandavasu, O., & Wexler, I. Withdrawal symptoms in infants with the fetal alcohol syndrome. *Pediatrics*, 1977, *90*, 630-633.

Priestly, B.L. Neurological assessment of infants of diabetic mothers in the first week of life. *Pediatrics*, 1972, *50*, 578-583.

Rubin, R.A., Rosenblatt, C. & Barlow, B. Psychological and educational sequelae of prematurity. *Pediatrics*, 1973, *52*, 352-363.

Rush, D. Examination of the relationship between birthweight, cigarette smoking during pregnancy and meternal weight gain. *Journal of Obstetrics and Gynecology, British Commonwealth*, 1974, *81*, 746-752.

Schafer, A.I. Teratogenic effects of antileukemic chemotherapy. *Archives of Internal Medicine*, 1981, *141*, 514-515.

Shurtleff, C.F., & Shurtleff, D.B. Environmental causes of birth defects. In K.I. Abrums & J.W. Bennett (Eds.), *Issues in genetics and exceptional children*. San Francisco: Jossey-Bass, 1981.

Simpson, W.J.A. A preliminary report on cigarette smoking and the incidence of prematurity. *American Journal of Obstetrics and Gynecology*, 1957, *73*, 808.

Smith, D.W. The fetal alcohol syndrome. *Hospital Practice*, 1979, *14*(10), 121-128.

Smith, D.W. *Recognizable patterns of human malformation* (3rd ed.) New York: Grune & Stratton, 1982.

Sokol, R.J., Miller, S.I., & Martier, S.S. *Preventing fetal alcohol effects: a practical guide for ob/gyn physicians and nurses*. Washington, DC: National Institute on Alcohol Abuse and Alcoholism, 1982.

Soler, N.G., Walsh, C.H., & Malins, J.M. Congenital malformations in infants of diabetic mothers. *Quarterly Journal of Medicine*, 1976, *45*, 303-313.

Sparks, S. Speech and language in fetal alcohol syndrome, *Asha. Journal of the American Speech Language Hearing Association*,1984.

Spense, A.A., Cohen, E.N., & Brown, B.W., Jr. Occupational hazards for operating room based physicians. *Journal of the American Medical Association*, 1977, *283*, 955.

Spielberg, S.P. Pharmacogenetics and the fetus, *New England Journal of Medicine*, 1982, *307*(2), 115-116.

Spiers, P.S. Does growth retardation predespose the fetus to congenital malformations? *Lancet*, 1982, *2*, 312-314.

Stehbens, J.A., Baker, G.L., & Kitchell, M. Outcome at ages 1, 3, and 5 years of children born to diabetic women. *American Journal Obstetrics and Gynecology*, 1977, *127*(4), 408-413.

Stein, Z.A., & Susser, M.W. Prenatal nutrition and mental competence. In J. Lloyd-Still (Ed.), *Malnutrition and intellectual development*. Lancaster, England: MTP Press, 1976.

Stewart, A.L., Reynolds, E.O.R., & Lipscomb, A.P. Outcome for infants of very low birthweight: Survey of world literature. *Lancet*, 1981, *1*, 1038-1040.

Streissguth, A.P., Herman, C.S., & Smith, D.W. Intelligence, behavior and dysmorphogenesis in the fetal alcohol syndrome: A report on 20 patients. *Journal of Pediatrics*, 1978, 92(3), 363-367.

Streissguth, A.P., Landesman-Dwyer, S., Martin, J.C., & Smith, D.W. Teratogenic effects of alcohol in humans and laboratory animals. *Science*, 1980, *209*, 353-361.

Strobino, B.R., Kline, J. & Stein, Z. Clinical and physical exposure of parents; Effect on human reproduction and offspring. *Journal of Human Development*, 1978, *1*, (4), 371-399.

Taylor, D.C. Differential rates of cerebral maturation between sexes and between hemispheres. *Lancet*, 1969, 2, 140-142.

Thompson, J.S., & Thompson, M.W. *Genetics in medicine* (3rd ed.) Philadelphia: Saunders, 1980.

Vetter, D.K., Fay, W.H., & Winitz, H. In F.M. Lassman, R.O. Fisch, D.K. Vetter et al. (Eds.) *Early correlates of speech, language, and hearing* (pp.266-329). Littleton, MA: PSG Publishing, 1980.

Vorhees, C.V., Brunner, R.L., & Butcher, R.E. Psychotropic drugs as behavioral teratogens. *Science*, 1979, *205*, 1220-1225.

Wada, J.A., Clarke, R., & Hamm, A. Cerebral hemispheric asymmetry in humans. Cortical speech zones in 100 adults and 100 infant brains. *Archives of Neurology*, 1975, *32*, 239-246.

Wilson, G.S., McCreary,R., Kean, J., & Baxter, J.C. The development of preschool children of heroin addicted mothers: A controlled study. *Pediatrics*, 1979, *63*, 135-141.

Winick, M. *Malnutrition and brain development*. New York: Oxford University Press, 1976.

Winick, M., & Noble, A. Cellular response in rats during malnutrition at various ages. *Journal of Nutrition*, 1966, 89, 300.

Witelson, S.J., & Pallie, W. Left hemisphere specialization for language in the newborn: Neuroanatomical evidence of asymmetry. *Brain*, 1973, 96, 641-647.

Wolff, P.H. Critical periods in human cognitive development. *Hospital Practice*, 1970, 5, 77-87.

Yogman, M.W., Cole, P., Als, H., & Lester, B.M. Behavior of newborns of diabetic mothers. *Infant Behavior & Development*, 1982, 5(4), 331-340.

6
Perinatal and Iatrogenic Birth Defects

Thus far the birth defects addressed have had prenatal origins, either genetic or environmental. Some birth defects are caused by injuries to the newborn during the time that surrounds the birth process, which is known as the *perinatal* period. If it is assumed that injury to the central nervous system may in turn place a child at risk for language and speech problems, clinicians must be concerned with perinatal birth defects. *Iatrogenic* birth defects are the result of treatment used to maintain the life of the newborn. Clinicians may play an important part in the prevention of some iatrogenic birth defects.

PERINATAL CAUSES OF BIRTH DEFECTS

Problems during labor and delivery account for 20% of still births, 20 to 40% on cerebral palsy, and 10% of severe mental retardation (Committee on Perinatal Health, 1976). The central and peripheral nervous systems of the fetus and neonate are at risk in the perinatal period from asphyxia, obstetrical trauma, and anesthetic intoxication (Painter, 1979). Furthermore, as Prechtl and Beintema (1964) noted, problems during delivery are usually not isolated events. While the occurrence of a single adverse incident during delivery may have little effect on behavior, multiple incidents may result in central nervous system injury and may increase the risk of later abnormal outcome.

Asphyxia

Brain damage in the perinatal period is most often caused by those conditions that lead to oxygen deprivation to the susceptible brain cells, a condition known as asphyxia or anoxia. Interruption of the oxygen supply to the fetus during the time of birth is perinatal asphyxia. A neonate is classified as having been asphyxiated if bag-and-mask resuscitation is required for over 1 minute in the delivery room. The incidence of asphyxia is 1 in 13,000 deliveries (Painter, 1979). Only a fraction of these are in danger of permanent damage.

Some conditions in the mother predispose a neonate to asphyxia: (a) eclampsia, a convulsive seizure brought on by toxemia (a disturbance of maternal metabolism with water retention and hypertension); (b) preeclampsia, a state of toxemia without convulsions; (c) diabetes; (d) anemia; and (e) hypotension or decreased blood pressure. Two conditions of delivery also place an infant at high risk for asphyxia (Dorand, 1977): placenta previa, (the placenta is over or immediately adjacent to the uterine cervix, which produces serious hemorrhage during delivery); and abruptio placenta (premature separation of the placenta from the uterus before delivery of the fetus).

Asphyxia during delivery may be acute and total or, more commonly, a prolonged and partial decrease of oxygen to the neonate. Complete and total asphyxia can occur when the umbilical cord is clamped or compressed, as when the fetus is in breech position (the presentation of the buttocks first in delivery) and at greatest risk for injury to the central nervous system. Prolonged, partial asyphxia can be produced by very strong uterine contractions during delivery (Painter, 1979). The site of the brain damage that can result from the lack of oxygen primarily involves the cerebral hemispheres. Although the reasons are not understood, the left temporal lobe is particularly vulnerable to insult at birth in boys (Ferry, Culbertson, Fitzgibbons, & Netsky, 1979). Boys are also known to have a higher incidence of language problems and learning disabilities than girls (Goldman, 1975), which could be related to temporal lobe damage.

When the cerebral cortex has been damaged from lack of oxygen, alterations in muscle tone are commonly noted. In premature infants, marked hypotonia may be evident in the legs. In the full-term infant, the clinical picture of hypotonia varies, and the degree of severity is of prognostic significance (Painter, 1979). Brown, Purvis, Forfar, & Cockburn (1974) noted that the longer the hypotonia persisted, the more ominous the outlook for development. The presence of hypotonia is clinically significant in the evaluation for speech and language (see Appendices).

Cerebral palsy has long been known to be associated with perinatal asphyxia (D'Souza & Richards, 1978; Scott, 1976;

Thompson, Searle, & Russell, 1977), but most children surviving severe perinatal asphyxia do so without severe mental or physical handicaps. The role that perinatal asphyxia plays in speech and language disorders is not clear. D'Souza, McCartney, Nolan, & Taylor (1981) assessed the speech and language of a group of 24 children in England who had been asphyxiated for at least 10 minutes at birth. Two had severe physical handicaps, but one third of the children without serious mental or physical handicaps had deficits in speech and language. The children were evaluated on The Reynell Developmental Language Scales, which yielded verbal comprehension and expressive language scales. Although no reference for the test was given, this study warrants scrutiny because a speech and language evaluation instrument was used. Results were given for the 5 children of the 24 whose language scores were below one standard deviation from the mean. Two of the 5 had receptive and expressive language delay "for no known reason," 1 was classified as mentally impaired, 1 had arrested hydrocephalus and 1 had depressed hearing on that day. Of the 3 who had articulation defects, one also had delayed verbal comprehension and one had above-age-level verbal comprehension. Curiously, no expressive language scores were given for those 3 cases. Although cause and effect cannot be established without further studies, it would appear that the child who survives severe perinatal asphyxia is at risk for speech and language delay even in the absence of physical symptoms and should be evaluated.

Obstetrical Trauma

Although the risk of injury due to obstetrical trauma is greatly reduced from former times, these injuries do occur. The infant at greatest risk for injury to any part of the central nervous system is the infant in breech presentation. It is even more dangerous for premature infants delivered in breech presentation (Goldenberg & Nelson, 1977). High incidence of asphyxia and cerebral hemorrhage associated with the delivery of the head occurs in this group. Babies who are known to be in breech position are likely to be delivered by cesarean section to avoid the high risks of breech delivery. Perinatal brain damage may also be the result of injury to blood vessels in the brain and consequent bleeding. Again, infants in breech presentation are 10 times more likely to have subdural hematomas (blood clots due to bleeding from ruptured blood vessels) than those born in head-first presentation (Abroms, McLennan & Mandell, 1977). Large infants of mothers having their first baby and infants who are delivered rapidly of mothers who have had multiple deliveries are at risk for developing a subdural hemorrhage.

Anesthetic Intoxication

Anesthetic agents given to the laboring mother may affect the fetus. Any agent that produces maternal hypotension may decrease the gas exchange between mother and fetus, resulting in reduction of oxygen to the fetus, which, in turn, may damage the brain. The evidence is inconclusive on the merits of local versus sedative anesthesia and their effects on behavorial responses of the infant (Corke, 1977; Scanlon, 1974). Oversedation in the mother may result in reduced oxygen to the fetus. Although local anesthetics decrease the number of sedative and narcotic agents administered to the mother, they also are absorbed by the mother and may cross the placenta to affect the fetus.

Seizures

Seizures in a child's perinatal history should alert the clinician to potential problems, but the timing of the seizures is important. Seizures can be a sign of increased intracranial pressure, such as in subdural hematoma (Painter, 1979). Seizures occurring within the first 4 days are often the result of brain damage and anoxia. However, seizures occurring initially toward the end of the 1st week and into the 2nd week of life frequently have a metabolic etiology, in which case the prognosis for normal development is good (Knauss & Marshall, 1977).

Kernicterus

Hyperbilirubinemia occurs in the newborn when an excess of serum bilirubin is present in the infant's blood and is evident by the presence of jaundice. Bilirubin is normally excreted by the newborn through the liver and urine without harm. If bilirubin is not excreted, it can result in the condition of kernicterus, which is characterized by severe jaundice and may be accompanied by poor feeding, lethargy, depressed Moro reflex (primitive startle reflex), unusual posturing, high-frequency-hearing loss, ataxia, choreoathetosis (involuntary movements of both chorea and athetosis), and seizures. If not treated, this disorder can result in mental retardation or death. Kernicterus generally occurs when concentrations of bilirubin in the blood exceed 20 to 25 mg per 100 ml (Telzrow, Snyder, Tronick, Als, & Brazelton, 1980).

The most frequent treatment for mild cases of neonatal jaundice with bilirubin levels of 13 to 14 mg%, is phototherapy in which the infant is placed under fluorescent lights. Severe cases require exchange transfusions of blood. Although there is some evidence that even infants with mild cases treated with phototherapy show some behavioral differences from normal infants in the early weeks of life (Nelson & Horowitz, 1982), the persistence of those differences and the effect on cognition has not been sufficiently explored. The prevalence of physiologic jaundice in the newborn (50% of full-term infants and 80% of preterm infants) (Maisels, 1975) would argue that the condition itself is not handicapping. The clinician should be alert to evidence of the serious condition of kernicterus that may affect hearing, cognition, and neurodevelopment.

Case Report

Matthew was brought to the WMU Language, Speech and Hearing Clinic at age 2. He was a very social child who communicated well with gestures, but his expressive language consisted of the one word, "pop," and an occasional "mama." He walked at 22 months with a scissors gait and was obviously physically delayed. He began speech therapy, occupational therapy, and a special education class in the public school at age 2 1/2.

Matthew's mother reported a complex perinatal history. His birth weight was 5 lb 6 oz and length was 18 in. Matthew was born with the umbilical cord wrapped around his neck, and bag-and-mask rescusitation was needed for 8 minutes. The day after birth, he suffered 10 seizures within a period of 15 hours. Phenobarbital was administered for the seizures. Meconium (stool that collects in the intestine of the fetus and is usually not discharged until after birth) was found in the amniotic fluid, which indicated fetal stress. The physician reported that although Matthew was born 2 weeks after the expected birth date, the placenta may not have functioned well after 7 months. Inadequate nourishment could account for fetal stress, and he may have actually lost weight in utero.

Matthew's speech musculature, like his whole body, was hypotonic. Tongue motions were slow and unsure. His voice was weak and breathy. As he became verbal, his speech was slow and slurred, and he ran out of breath after only a few syllables. He remained at the one- and two-word level until he was nearly 4 years old; it seemed that he simply could not muster the strength to say more. When asked to increase his loudness level, he could shout a response, but there was no gradation of loudness. His early language consisted mostly of vowel sounds with omission of most consonants, especially in final position. The /h/ and /w/ sounds were especially difficult because of the breath expended for the first and the lip rounding for the second. In many ways, Matthew's uncoordinated movements were like those of oral apraxia. However, diagnostic evaluation revealed that his problem was not motor planning; it was severe hypotonia in his speech musculature. This diagnosis was consistent with his perinatal asphyxia.

Matthew's therapy consisted of strengthening all his speech muscles, beginning with those for breath control. He blew bubbles to increase his stamina, first through a straw into water and then through the small wire loop. Gradation of loudness was accomplished with a sound-intensity meter. Exercises for lip pursing and tongue mobility were also incorporated.

Matthew's receptive language remained at age level and above, and by age 4 1/2 he began to express himself in sentences at a very slow rate. His language was syntactically correct, but he still seemed to shorten his utterances to conserve his breath supply. He was considerably smaller than other children his age, and his parents planned to enroll him in regular kindergarten at age 6 along with continuous speech therapy and occupational therapy. Although it appeared that his was a case of delayed language, his speech problems proved to be entirely motor. Goals, therefore, were focused on intensive therapy for the motor processes of speech and increased muscle tone.

IATROGENIC BIRTH DEFECTS

It is now widely accepted that the introduction of the Neonatal Intensive Care Unit (NICU) in hospitals has increased infant survival rates because of sophisticated technology and improved techniques employed by attending personnel (Teberg, Hodgman, Wu, & Spears, 1977; Paneth et al., 1982; Stewart, Reynolds, & Lipscomb, 1981).

The primary concern of medical professionals in the NICU is to sustain the life of the infant. The long-term side effects of that treatment have been a secondary consideration. However, it is the responsibility of professionals, including clinicians, to identify these long-term side effects and habilitate or rehabilitate the affected children.

Three iatrogenic (treatment-induced) conditions are of primary concern to the clinician: voice disorders from endotracheal intubation; aphonia from tracheostomy; and hearing loss from con-ditions in the NICU.

Voice Disorders from Endotracheal Intubation

Although various types of injury to newborns can be caused by instrumentation, injury from intubation is still by far the most common (Richardson, 1981.) An endotracheal tube may be placed in the airway of a neonate who is incapable of breathing in-dependently due to respiratory distress (Hawkins, 1978; Joshi, Mandavia, Stern, & Wiglesworth, 1972; Parkin, Stevens, & Jung, 1976). As Otherson (1979) notes: "Ventilatory support by endotracheal tube is almost a routine procedure in newborn respiratory distress, in the postoperative period and in the therapy of any acute illness or injury. In fact, these tubes in the airway have become so common that they are frequently not treated with the proper regard and respect" (p.601). The tube goes through the larynx and may produce injury when it is placed initially or after prolonged intubation.

The leading cause of intubation injury is an endotracheal tube that is too large for the trachea. The anatomic dimensions of the airway in infants invite the insertion of an endotracheal tube that is too large and fits too snugly. In infants, the cricoid ring is the narrowest section of the airway, and a tube that appears to fit easi-ly through the glottis of an infant may be too tight in the cricoid and could produce pressure necrosis (tissue death). Tapered tubes may also be damaging; when inserted and advanced into the trachea, the enlarged portion of the tube impinges on the vocal folds and may produce pressure necrosis (Otherson, 1979).

Besides the fit of the tube, there are some other causes of laryngeal damage from intubation: (a) Infections may result from placement. If the mucosa is lacerated at the time of intubation, an avenue for bacterial invasion of submucosal tissues is opened. (b) Respirator tubing is heavy, and when unsupported it tugs on the endotracheal tube, causing mucosal swelling. (c) The tube which has a gradually curving shape known as the McGill design, puts significant pressure on the posterior commissure from the weight of the tongue resting on the tube. (d) The posterior commissure and arytenoid area is a triangular anatomic space that is filled with a round tube. Inappropriate matching of shapes subjects several areas in the larynx to injury, especially the vocal processes of the arytenoids and the midline of the posterior commissure. Round grooves can be produced in the vocal processes that lead to incomplete glottic closure and breathy voice. (e) Excessive pressure induced by the endotracheal cuff of the tube may cause damage to the delicate tissues of the mucosa and tracheal wall.

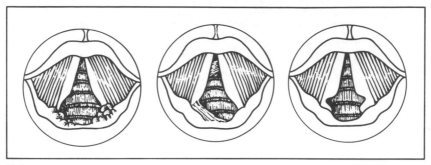

FIGURE 6-1
From "Injuries to the neonatal larynx from long term endotracheal tube intubation and suggested tube modification for prevention" by A.S. Hengerer, M. Strome, & B.F. Jaffe, *Annals of Otology, Rhinology and Laryngology*, 1975, 84, 764-770. Reprinted by permission.

Vocal pathology

Many authors have described laryngeal damage from intubation (Joshi et al., 1972; McGovern, Fitz-Hugh, & Edgemon, 1971; Parkin et al., 1976; Richardson, 1981). The most serious complication of endotracheal intubation is laryngeal stenosis. Anterior webbing between the vocal folds may develop as a result of irritation from the tube. The vocal folds are the commonest lesion sites, with or without extension of the lesions to the subglottic region of the larynx and trachea. Two accounts described the vocal characteristics of the children after intubation. Hawkins (1978) found hoarseness in a few cases and Hengerer, Strome, and Jaffe (1975) described four cases of children from 6 months to 3 years old with hoarse and breathy voices.

Prevention

Modifications for intubation equipment to prevent injury have been suggested by Hengerer et al., (1975); Otherson, (1979); Stewart, Finer, Moriartey, & Ulan (1980); McGovern et al., (1971) and Lewis, Schlobohm, & Thomas (1978): (a) A triangular section of the tube may decrease the grooving process at the posterior commissure and arytenoid area. (b) Uniform-diameter soft polyvinyl tubing with a reverse curve and the smallest tube size should be chosen to decrease the amount of pressure on the vocal tract. (c) Taping the tube securely to limit the piston action transmitted from the respirator will decrease ulcerations. (d) Adequate hydration is necessary to help prevent drying of the secretions on the tube and the membranes adjacent to it.

Stewart et al., (1980) note that complications following intubation may be prevented when certain precautions are observed. (a) Endotracheal intubation should be administered by an experienced practitioner, the endotracheal tube stabilized firmly, and rigid technique of tube care observed. (b) Standard elective tube changes should be avoided. (c) Ventilation should be low pressure if possible. (d) Safe and skilled extubation technique is required.

The clinician may incorrectly assume that the NICU staff is well aware of iatrogenic injury from intubation. Members of the NICU staff are not the professionals most concerned with voice disorders. Here, as in the following sections, the clinician has an opportunity to prevent disorders by educating other health professionals.

Aphonia from Tracheostomy

While endotracheal intubation may be the primary treatment for establishing an airway, the infant in the NICU may require a *tracheostomy* on a long-term basis for continued ventilation. A tracheostomy is an artificial opening from the neck into the trachea. A tube (cannula) is placed in the opening to provide an airway in cases in which the airway is blocked due to tracheal stenosis or other obstruction, or in cases of severe respiratory distress, which require suctioning (Ross, 1982; Simon & Handler, 1981). As the child breathes or is assisted by a ventilator, air is delivered directly to the lungs. If the tracheostomy tube fits snugly inside the trachea, all the air will go in and out of the tube, and there is no air channeled upward for phonation through the larynx. However, if there is a leak in the tube from a space between the tube and the trachea, or if there is an opening (fenestration) cut into the top of the tube, expired air can pass up through the glottis and the vocal folds and allow vocalization.

The use of the mechanical ventilator also places certain restrictions on the rate of swallowing and breathing and affects attempts to vocalize. Some children may actually vocalize more easily on inspiration, which may prove confusing to the child when he is gradually weaned away from the ventilator. There is a high incidence of otitis media in these patients; perhaps the swallowing patterns contribute to eustachean tube dysfunction with middle ear fluid as a result.

Role of the Clinician in Tracheostomy

Cases have been reported in which the cannula was not removed until the child was well over 3 years old, during which time there was no opportunity to emit normal speech sounds (Ross, 1982). This poses some unique problems for the clinician, some of which can be prevented with the cooperation of the NICU personnel.

The clinician's role begins with the child in the hospital and involves evaluation, therapy, and education and counseling for the parents and hospital personnel. If the infant will have a tracheostomy tube for a short period of time, the involvement of the clinician is not warranted; those children with an expected duration of tracheostomy for longer than 2 to 3 weeks should be assessed. (Simon & Handler, 1981).

Evaluation

After the general case history information is obtained, the assessment of communication skills will begin with assessment of the ability to produce voice and under what conditions voice is possible. It may be that voice can only occur when the child is in a certain body position or when he lowers his head to block the tube. Can voice be emitted when the child is on the ventilator? The quality and intensity of the voice should also be noted. What is the child's means of expressive language? If voice is absent, what is the cause of the inability to vocalize? Is it the tight-fitting tube, interference from the ventilator, or a condition in the trachea or larynx? What are the conditions of the oral-motor reflexes and their functioning for speech and feeding? Finally, the clinician should note the child's ability in receptive language with an assessment instrument, such as the REEL (Receptive, Expressive Emergent Language Scale, Bzoch & League, 1971). The parent will be the informant for the history and the receptive language assessment.

Therapy

Therapy consists of voice production if possible, language and speech stimulation, and oral facilitation to decrease abnormal oral reflexes and improve skills for oral feeding. Therapy should begin at the bedside with attempts to stimulate language while nurses are changing or bathing the child. It is important to initiate therapy in the child's crib with his own toys so that he does not feel threatened. The clinician will not be welcome in the NICU unless he or she scrupulously abides by the rules of sterile or sanitary conditions.

The clinician must also become familiar with the equipment and ways to position the patient, while watching for changes in the patient that necessitate help from the nurses.

Voice production

The clinician should determine the child's ability to phonate either naturally, from leaked air into the glottis, or manually, by occluding the tracheostomy briefly with the finger. If this produces voice, the child can be taught to occlude the tube or depress his chin to vocalize. Some tracheostomized children often display ingenuity in vocal communication without being formally taught: self-taught esophageal speech, lingual clicks and pops, breath sounds, and lip movements, as well as the ability to phonate by putting the chin down to displace the tracheal tube, have been reported (Ross, 1982).

Tracheostomized children with neuromuscular disorders may not have the muscle strength or coordination to accomplish speech production and may need to develop their muscles of respiration before vocalization is possible. These children may have been fed through nasogastric or gastrostomy tubes and consequently may not have received oral stimulation from feeding experiences that help to develop speech. As a result, when the tracheostomy is removed (decannulation) they may be hypersensitive around the mouth and have a hypersensitive gag reflex (Simon & Handler, 1981).

Language

If there is not enough air leakage around the tube for vocalization, manual language can be taught to nonvocal children. The parents should be reassured that signing will fade away when the child is vocal but that a symbol system aids development by allowing the child to use expressive language (Simon, Fowler, & Handler, 1982).

The effect that aphonia from long-term tracheostomy has on language development has not been investigated adequately. Ross (1982) studied the language of six boys from 32 to 46 months of age who had tracheal tubes from 11 to 44 months. All six produced voice after decannulation. These children did not babble or have the opportunity to practice speech and yet, when decannulated, a few of the children passed through each normal stage of expressive language, with the exception of babbling, at an accelerated pace until their syntactic development reached age level. Ross concluded that the language development of the children was more dependent upon the intellectual functioning of the child than upon the length of aphonia. Cognitive ability could be impaired due to the perinatal problems that required the tracheostomy and that impairment appears to have a more serious effect on lanugage than the lack of opportunity to produce speech. These results suggest that it is not necessary to vocalize in order to develop normal speech as long as sufficient language is heard during the aphonic period.

Oral-motor facilitation

The child who is tube fed may be given the experience of sucking on a pacifier for oral stimulation while he is taking nourishment. The clinician can create more enjoyable feeding sessions for the child by encouraging the nursing staff and family to hold the infant while he or she is fed (Simon & Handler, 1981).

Education and prevention

Physicians may lack interest in the speech development of these children for a number of reasons: (a) Tracheostomy is usually of short duration. (b) Many children can phonate around the tube. (c) The physician is preoccupied with the severe medical problems of these children. (d) Physicians mistakenly assume that speech therapy is difficult with these children and that the child will speak immediately when the tube is taken out (Simon et al., 1982). The clinician should work with the physician to find a way to facilitate air leakage into the glottis; perhaps a smaller tube or one that fits less snugly will work as well for the required ventilation. The clinician can educate the hospital staff and parents about the importance of language development, feeding techniques, ways to decrease abnormal oral reflexes, and methods of stimulating verbal and nonverbal language.

The importance of receptive language stimulation while the child is in the hospital should be stressed to the parents. If the child is sent home with the tracheostomy tube in place, the parents will assume the major responsibility for home therapy with help from the clinician. Some children go to school with tracheostomies and the clinician may first encounter them there or in home visits. When the child is decannulated, therapy may be directed toward language development and improving intelligibility (Simon & Handler, 1981).

Iatrogenic Hearing Loss

Noise levels in the NICU as a cause of hearing loss have been studied extensively (Douek, Banister, Dodson, Ashcroft & Humphries, 1976; Long, Lucey, & Philip, 1980). The incidence of hearing loss in infants is 1 in 50 when neonates have been cared for in an NICU. The continuous nature of the noise, which does not allow time for recovery, may cause damage to the immature cochlea.

A risk register for neonates was developed by a Joint Committee on Hearing Screening (Northern & Downs, 1974). Five factors are considered in this register, and an infant having any one of the five is assumed to be at risk: (a) family history of childhood deafness; (b) maternal rubella during pregnancy or other intrauterine viral infection; (c) hyperbilirubinemia; (d) maxillofacial anomalies; and (e) prematurity or birth weight of 1,500 g (5 lb) or less. Two more neonatal conditions should be added (Poland, Wells, & Ferlauto, 1980): severe perinatal anoxia and metabolic acidosis (lowered pH of the blood). Treatment with drugs that are known to be ototoxic also places a neonate at risk for hearing loss: salicylates and quinine; potent diuretics; certain anticancer drugs; and some antibiotics (streptomycin, kanamycin, neomycin, gentamicin, and tobramycin) (Falk, 1972; Golbus, 1980).

Causes of high noise levels in the NICU

Long, Lucey, and Philip (1980) found equipment in the NICU (cardiac monitors, the capillary tube centrifuge, and the telephone) to be the greatest noise offenders, although staff noise contributed also. Hospital incubators accounted for noise levels between 50 and 86 dB. They also found the incubators to muffle some external noises; outside the incubator, the levels were 55 to 75 dB, while inside, noise levels were 50 to 57 dB SPL. Average noise levels from staff activity (closing doors and drawers, laughter, and conversation) were at 60 to 65 dB with deflections into the 70 to 75 dB range. Slamming of incubator doors and crying infants can produce up to 90 to 100 dB.

A recent investigation by D'Souza et al. (1981) throws some doubt on the common belief that ototoxic drugs and incubator noise have a synergistic effect. Twenty-six babies received gentamicin and incubator care for an average of 8 days following severe perinatal asphyxia. The noise level in the incubator was 67 dB with alarms peaking to 78 dB. Only one of the babies was found to have a sensorineural hearing loss. This incidence of 4% is the same as the incidence of sensorineural deafness in survivors of severe perinatal asphyxia. However, until this study has been duplicated, precautions against high-noise-level damage should be maintained.

Prevention of hearing loss in the NICU

If hearing loss can be caused by high noise levels in the NICU, the incidence of loss should be alleviated by lowering those noise levels. Long et al. (1980) asked an NICU staff to reduce their noise-producing activities. The systolic "beep" on the cardiac monitors was silenced, the centrifuge was removed, and the telephones were muffled. These measures reduced the noise levels from 60 to 65 dB to a slightly lower baseline (58 to 63 dB), but with deflections as great as the previous baseline. When the staff reduced their own noise-producing activities, (laughter, loud conversation, banging drawers, etc.) noise levels within the incubators fell to 50 to 57 dB. The investigators concluded that professionals working in the NICU should pay more attention to an important source of noise pollution, themselves.

In 1974, the American Academy of Pediatrics Committee on Environmental Hazards suggested prevention of noise-induced trauma through measures similar to those of the Long et al. (1980) study: (a) Incubator manufacturers should lower motor noise levels; (b) physicians should limit the use of ototoxic drugs as much as possible; and (c) hospital personnel should limit unnecessary noise. The speech-language clinician and audiologist in the hospital should take the lead in bringing this to the attention of the NICU staff.

REFERENCES

Abroms, I.F., McLennan, J.E., & Mandell, F. Acute neonatal subdural hematoma following breech delivery. *American Journal of Diseases of Children,* 1977, *131,* 192-194.

American Academy of Pediatrics Committee on Environmental Hazards. Noise pollution: Neonatal aspects. *Pediatrics,* 1974, *54,* 476-479.

Brown, J.K., Purvis, R.J., Forfar, J.O., & Cockburn, F. Neurological aspects of perinatal asphyxia. *Developmental Medicine and Child Neurology,* 1974, *16,* 567-580.

Bzoch, K.R., & League, R. *Receptive Expressive Emergent Language Scale.* Baltimore: University Park Press, 1971.

Committee on Perinatal Health. *Toward improving the outcome of pregnancy: Recommendations for the regional development of maternal and perinatal health services.* White Plains, NY: The National Foundation-March of Dimes, 1976.

Corke, B.C. Neurobehavioral responses of the newborn: The effect of different forms of maternal analgesia. *Anesthesia,* 1977, *32,* 539.

Dorand, R.D. Neonatal asphyxia. An approach to physiology and management. *Pediatric Clinics of North America,* 1977, *24,* 455.

Douek, E., Banister, L.H., Dodson, H.C., Ashcroft, P., & Humphries, K.N. Effects of incubator noise on the cochlea of the newborn. *Lancet,* 1976, *2,* 1110-1113.

D'Souza, S.W., McCartney, E., Nolan, M., & Taylor, I.G. Hearing, speech, and language in survivors of severe perinatal asphyxia. *Archives of Disease in Childhood,* 1981, *56,* 245-252.

D'Souza, S.W., & Richards, B. Neurological sequelae in newborn babies after perinatal asphyxia. *Archives of Disease in Childhood,* 1978, *53,* 564-569.

Falk, S.A. Combined effects of noise and ototoxic drugs. *Environmental Health Perspective,* 1972, *2,* 5-22.

Ferry, P.C., Culbertson, J.L., Fitzgibbons, P.M., & Netsky, M.G. Brain function and language disabilities. *International Journal of Pediatric Otorhinolaryngology,* 1979, *1,* 13-24.

Golbus, M.S. Teratology for the obstetrician: Current status. *Obstetrics and Gynecology,* 1980, *55*(3), 1-9.

Goldenberg, R.L., & Nelson, K. The premature breech. *American Journal of Obstetrics and Gynecology,* 1977, *127,* 240.

Goldman, P.S. Age, sex and experience as related to the neural basis of cognitive development. In N.A. Buchwald & M.A. Brazier (Eds.), *Brain mechanisms in mental retardation* (Chapter 13). New York: Academic Press, 1975.

Hawkins, D.B. Hyaline membrane disease of the neonate. Prolonged intubation in management: Effects on the larynx. *Laryngoscope,* 1978, *88,* 201-224.

Hengerer, A.S., Strome, M., & Jaffe, B.F. Injuries to the neonatal larynx from long term endotracheal tube intubation and suggested tube modification for prevention. *Annals of Otology, Rhinology and Laryngology,* 1975, *84,* 764-770.

Joshi, V.V., Mandavia, S.G., Stern, L., & Wiglesworth, F.W. Acute lesions induced by endotracheal intubation. *American Journal of Diseases of Children,* 1972, *124,* 646-649.

Knauss, T.A., & Marshall, R.E. Seizures in a neonatal intensive care unit. *Developmental Medicine and Child Neurology,* 1977, *19,* 719-728.

Lewis, F.R., Schlobohm, R.M., & Thomas, A.N. Prevention of complications from prolonged tracheal intubation. *American Journal of Surgery,* 1978, *135,* 453-457.

Long, J.G., Lucey, J.F., & Philip, A.G.S. Noise and hypoxemia in the intensive care nursery. *Pediatrics,* 1980, *65,* 143-145.

Maisels, M.M. Neonatal jaundice. In G.B. Avery (Ed.), *Neonatology: Pathophysiology and management of the newborn.* Philadelphia: Lippincott, 1975.

McGovern, F.A., Fitz-Hugh, G.S., & Edgemon, L.J. The hazards of endotracheal intubation. *Annals of Otology, Rhinology, and Laryngology,* 1971, 80, 556-563.

Nelson, C.A., & Horowitz, F.D. The short-term sequelae of neonatal jaundice treated with phototherapy. *Infant Behavior & Development,* 1982, 5(3), 289-299.

Northern, J.L., & Downs, M.P. *Hearing in children.* Baltimore: Williams & Williams, 1974.

Otherson, H.B. Intubation injuries of the trachea in children. *Annals of Surgery,* 1979, 5, 601-606.

Painter, M.J. Neurologic sequalae of birth. In J.J. Sciarria (Ed.), *Gynecology and obstetrics:* Vol. 3 (Chapter 99). Hagerstown, MD: Harper & Row, 1979.

Paneth, N., Kiely, J.L., Phil, M., Wallenstein, S., Marcus, M., Pakter, J., & Susser, M. Newborn intensive care and neonatal mortality in low birth weight infants. *New England Journal of Medicine,* 1982. 307, 149-155.

Parkin, J.L., Stevens, M.H., & Jung, A.L. Acquired and congenital subglottic stenosis in the infant. *Annals of Otology, Rhinology and Laryngology,* 1976, 85, 573-581.

Poland, R.M., Wells, D.H., & Ferlauto, J.J. Methods for detecting hearing impairment in infancy. *Pediatric Annals,* 1980, 9(1), 31-44.

Prechtl, H., & Beintema, D. *The neurological examination of the full-term infant.* London: Heinemann, 1964.

Richardson, M.A. Laryngeal anatomy and mechanisms of trauma. *Ear, Nose, Throat Journal,* 1981, 60, 346-351.

Ross, G.S. Language functioning and speech development of six children receiving tracheotomy in infancy. *Journal of Communication Disorders,* 1982, 15, 95-111.

Scanlon, J.W. Neurobehavioral responses of newborn infants after maternal epidural anesthesia. *Anesthesiology,* 1974, 40, 121.

Scott, H. Outcome of very severe asphyxia. *Archives of Disease in Childhood,* 1976, 51, 712-716.

Simon, B., Fowler, S., & Handler, S.D. *Comprehensive management of communication needs for tracheostomized infants and children.* Paper presented to the American Speech-Language Hearing Association, Toronto, Canada, November, 1982.

Simon, B., & Handler, S.D. The speech pathologist and management of children with tracheostomies. *Journal of Otolaryngology,* 1981, 10, 440-448.

Stewart, A.L., Reynolds, E.O.R., & Lipscomb, A.P. Outcome for infants of very low birthweight: Survey of world literature. *Lancet,* 1981, 2, 1038-1040.

Stewart, A.R., Finer, N.N., Moriartey, R.R., & Ulan, O.A. Neonatal nasotracheal intubation: An evaluation. *Laryngoscope,* 1980, 90, 826-831.

Teberg, A., Hodgman, J.E., Wu, P.Y.K., & Spears, R.L. Recent improvement in outcome for the small premature infant. *Clinical Pediatrics,* 1977, 16, 307-313.

Telzrow, R.W., Snyder, D.M., Tronick, E., Als, H., & Brazelton, T.B. The behavior of jaundiced infants undergoing phototherapy. *Developmental Medicine and Child Neurology*, 1980, 22, 317-326.

Thompson, A.J., Searle, M., & Russell, G. Quality of survival after severe birth asphyxia. *Archives of Disease in Childhood*, 1977, 52, 620-626.

7

Genetic Counseling

Genetic counseling is a communication process that deals with the human problems associated with the occurrence, or the risk of occurrence, of a genetic disorder in a family. This process involves an attempt by one or more appropriately trained persons to help the individual or the family to (a) comprehend the medical facts, including the diagnosis, the probable course of the disorder, and the available management; (b) appreciate the way heredity contributes to the disorder and the risk of recurrence in specified relatives; (c) understand the options for dealing with the risk of recurrence; (d) choose the course of action that seems appropriate to them in view of their risk and their family goals and to act in accordance with that decision; and (e) make the best possible adjustment to the disorder in an affected family member and/or to the risk of recurrence of that disorder (Ad Hoc Committee on Genetic Counseling, 1975).

Principles of Genetic Counseling

The counseling process aims to help families through their problems, their decision making, their grief, and their adjustments. The goal is definitely not to make decisions for them. The first principle of genetic counseling is the neutrality of the counselor in decisions. Unlike the physician in the traditional role, who usually tells the patient what the treatment will be, the genetic counselor offers the patient information and possible options. This is unusual in medical practice. It is a difficult attitude for many physicians who do genetic counseling to adopt and may even be confusing to some patients, who expect to be guided by their physician (Porter, 1979). The second principle is that the information must be as accurate and complete as possible. Information must be in comprehensible terms, particularly when describing risk factors that involve percentages. Third, diagnosis of an affected child must be accurate. Failure to diagnose a birth defect, or misdiagnosis, has at least two serious consequences: it delays rehabilitation, and it prolongs the parents' confusion, anxiety, fear, and guilt. The family must know what the problems are before they can cope with them constructively. Too often, by the time a birth defect is diagnosed, the handicapped child may be in the first years of school.

Who Does Genetic Counseling?

Genetic counseling was begun by geneticists and physicians who were interested in genetics and thus working in departments or clinics not directly engaged in patient care. Therefore, genetic counseling developed from biological science rather than from clinical medicine (Porter, 1979). Index Medicus only began listing genetic counseling as a subject heading in 1973, reflecting the earlier lack of professional interest in this area (Weitz, 1981).

Currently, physicians in genetics are usually pediatricians, obstetricians/gynecologists, neurologists, or internists who have concentrated on genetic disorders. They often practice medicine in a major teaching hospital attached to a medical school (Milunsky, 1981). Those engaged in genetic counseling who are not physicians have usually earned graduate degrees in related fields, such as genetics or biochemistry.

Genetic counseling, like speech pathology in its early days, has a number of practitioners with divergent backgrounds. At the present time, there is no strict set of guidelines for training. The American Society of Human Genetics gave the first certifying examination in 1981 for peer certification. Those holding an academic degree of MD, PhD, or MS who take the examination must present credentials, including clinical and counseling experience. The examination covers basic genetics and human genetics, plus such specialty areas as cytogenetics, and counseling (G. Landenberger, personal communication, May, 1983). It is not a common area for a clinician to get an advanced degree, perhaps because of the lack of laboratory science necessary for the study of speech-language pathology. However, genetic counseling is a new and growing field with appeal for many who are also interested in human services.

Who Needs Genetic Counseling?

The reasons people seek genetic counseling can be grouped into five general categories. They want to know: (a) if they themselves have a genetic disorder or whether they are carriers for a genetic disorder; (b) if they have an increased risk of having a child (or another) affected with a particular genetic disorder; (c) what are the implications of a genetic disorder already diagnosed in an individual and what is the prognosis and treatment; (d) what help can they get in making a decision about the options of prenatal treatment, diagnosis, selective abortion, artificial insemination by donor, or adoption; and (e) what kind of help is available for their already affected child and where they can find it (Milunsky, 1977).

Indications for referral to genetic counseling

People may be referred to a genetic counselor if one of these conditions exists:

The Pregnant Couple:
   maternal age 35 or older
   paternal age 55 or older
   carriers of a known metabolic defect
   balanced translocation carrier
   previous child had a chromosomal defect
   previous child had a metabolic defect
   family history of neural tube defects, inherited disorder, or
      mental retardation of unknown etiology
   drug use or exposure to radiation or industrial chemicals.

The Couple That Has:
   lost a child with a known genetic disorder
   had two or more miscarriages
   been exposed to a potential teratogen or infectious agent
   had a stillborn child
   a positive family history of a genetic disorder.

The Child With:
   growth retardation
   mental retardation
   multiple congenital anomalies (dysmorphologies)
   muscular weakness
   neurological dysfunction
   bleeding tendencies
   a disorder of sexual development
   a metabolic disorder

Counseling is also recommended for individuals needing carrier testing; for example, hemophilia, muscular dystrophy, or chromosomal translocations.

Prenatal Diagnosis

In the late 1960's, advances in genetic medicine made it possible to detect before birth some disorders for which the fetus is at risk. Today prenatal detection is possible for most recognizable chromosomal anomalies, fetal-sex determination for the management of about 200 X-linked genetic disorders, over 100 biochemical genetic disorders, and open neural tube disorders. Over 60 autosomal recessive disorders are detectable prenatally, but there is only very rare detection of dominant genetic diseases (Golbus, 1982; Milunsky, 1981). Methods for detecting the absence or presence of these genetic defects prenatally include amniocentesis, diagnostic ultrasound, and fetoscopy.

Amniocentesis

Prenatal diagnosis actually became possible when amniocentesis was devised. Genetic counseling should be the preliminary step to amniocentesis. The counselor must record the family pedigree, verify medical history in relatives, determine which abnormalities are to be sought by amniocentesis, explain the procedure, and explore the patient's psychological reactions to both the procedure itself and to the information it might yield. If the couple wants to continue a known affected pregnancy, the value of amniocentesis is to prepare them for the birth of an affected child. It is crucial that the couple understands that amniocentesis rules out only specific diagnoses and that it is not a general test intended to screen for all possible abnormalities. A normal karyotype and test for neural tube defects from amniocentesis do not ensure a perfect baby.

Amniocentesis is done at about 14 to 16 weeks of pregnancy by an obstetrician. A sterile syringe is inserted through the mother's abdominal wall and into the uterus, which contains the amniotic fluid surrounding the fetus. About an ounce of amniotic fluid is withdrawn and transported to the genetics laboratory. Fetal cells in the amniotic fluid, sloughed off from the fetus, are cultured. Analyses are conducted for structure, number, and sex determination of the chromosomes (karyotype), and for neural tube defects. Screening for metabolic defects is more difficult and expensive; it is only done when indicated by a positive family history or a previous affected child (G. Landenberger, personal communication, May, 1983). The chromosomal diagnostic accuracy rate for amniocentesis is 99.4% (Pernoll, King & Prescott, 1980). Preliminary results of the chromosomal study can be obtained in about 16 days; metabolic studies take at least 1 to 6 weeks. This waiting interval is often emotionally trying for families, and they may need additional support during this interval. The overall risk of spontaneous abortion after amnioscentesis is less than 0.5% (Summer & Shoaf, 1982); the risk is dependent upon several factors, including the use of ultrasound and the experience of the physician who performs the procedure. There is no significant increased risk of fetal death, fetal injury, or complications of pregnancy after amniocentesis.

Indications for consideration of amniocentesis

(G. Landenberger, personal communication, May, 1983; McCormack, 1979; and Pernoll et al., 1980):

1. Maternal age of 35 years or older. Most amniocenteses are performed with advanced maternal age as the sole indication to exclude Down syndrome and other chromosomal disorders (see Chapter 2 for risk figures). The likelihood of diagnosing the disorder should be greater than the risk of amniocentesis.

2. Balanced translocation carrier parents. Most families in this category are detected only after the birth of a child with congenital anomalies due to an unbalanced translocation (see Chapter 1), or after experiencing several early miscarriages. Women undergoing amniocentesis when this is the reason for the procedure have a 10 to 15% incidence of abnormal fetuses. If the father is the carrier, the risk is only 5 to 7%.

3. Multiple pregnancy loss. Chromosomal anomalies in couples who have suffered three or more spontaneous abortions are about 12 times higher than in the general population.

4. Multiple congenital anomalies in previous offspring. The empiric risk of recurrence in most of these families, without a compounding history, is relatively low. However, anxiety concerning recurrence is often extremely high, and a couple may not attempt future pregnancy unless prenatal diagnosis is available.

5. Mother a known or presumed carrier of an X-linked recessive disorder. Women who are carriers for one of these conditions may undergo amniocentesis for the detection of the sex of the fetus. Although it cannot be determined if the condition is present in the fetus, a female child would have a 50% chance of being a carrier. A male child would have a 50% chance of being affected.

6. Previous child with a neural tube defect or first or second degree relative with a neural tube defect. Neural tube defects may be detected from elevated levels of alpha fetoprotein in the

amniotic fluid. The use of diagnostic ultrasound may improve the chance for diagnosis.

7. Both parents are carriers of a diagnosable autosomal recessive disorder on the basis of family history or previous screening tests. The couple may already have an affected child, or either parent may have an affected relative.

Diagnostic ultrasound

An image of the fetus (sonogram) is reflected onto a screen from high-frequency vibrations. Ultrasound can be used early in the 2nd trimester to measure the fetal skeleton and vital organs, including brain ventricles, heart, and kidneys. Routine ultrasound of every pregnancy in the 2nd trimester to assess gestational age and detect multiple fetuses has already been initiated in some centers and may become standard practice (Milunsky, 1981). Diagnostic ultrasound used prior to amniocentesis to detect anomalies and locate the placenta and parts of the fetus is more extensive than routine ultrasound.

Fetoscopy

Many genetic problems that cannot be diagnosed from amniotic fluid can be diagnosed by fetoscopy in which fetal blood and tissue samples are obtained. Guided by ultrasound, a fiberoptic scope (light source) is passed through the uterine wall. The fetoscope provides a limited opportunity to view the fetus for malformations. Tissue and blood are drawn through a cannula in the scope from the site of the insertion of the cord into the placenta. This procedure is done at only a few centers in the United States and has a 3% risk of inducing abortion (Golbus, 1982; G. Landenberger, personal communication, May, 1983).

Genetic and Newborn Screening

Genetic screening is a search for persons who possess certain genotypes that are already associated with a specific disorder or may lead to the disorder in their descendants (Abroms, 1981). One type of genetic screening is done to identify carriers for a specific genetic disorder and is done in those populations that have a high probability of carriers due to ethnic or geographical background in which certain genetic diseases are more prevalent, such as Tay-Sachs in persons of Ashkenazi Jewish background and sickle-cell anemia in the black population. A second type of screening, in the newborn, seeks to detect the presence of a genetic disease in its early stage in order to begin intervention for the prevention of symptoms, for example, phenylketonuria (PKU) and hypothyroidism (cretinism), disorders that cause mental retardation if left untreated. These screening tests may be done from blood and urine samples before the infant leaves the hospital.

Counseling Parents of Children with Birth Defects

Parents typically react to the discovery that their child has a birth defect as they would be expected to react to other tragic life events: with shock and disbelief. Grief for the loss of the anticipated perfect child and depression are followed by a phase of mourning, which help to prepare the parents for the eventual facing of reality and adaptive coping with the handicap. Little that is said to the parents immediately following the shock of the original diagnosis is remembered or assimilated by the parents. This is a very important principle to remember because physicians and counselors may go to great lengths to explain about rehabilitation when parents are emotionally unable to hear or understand the information (Vernon, 1979a). Parents who have suffered a fetal loss from miscarriage, stillbirth, or neonatal death have the same grief reactions (Standish, 1982). Those who deal with disordered children may also be dealing with some psychological defenses of their parents.

Anxiety

Even when the defect is not readily apparent prior to diagnosis, parents often sense that something is wrong and may feel a vague uneasiness. Anxiety increases as time passes and the child's lack of development becomes apparent. Once a physician is consulted, the parents may discuss their questions about the child's development. Some of these same concerns are also voiced by parents of normal children, and the physician may pass them off with assurances that the child will grow out of the problem or catch up. While such a response may temporarily allay concern, it eventually causes increasing frustration. The parents realize something is wrong but cannot communicate with their physician about it. "Doctor shopping," the endless series of consultations with health-care and counseling agencies, including speech and hearing centers, is common. Some parents become avid readers of medical literature and many are particularly vulnerable to quackery and poor counsel (Vernon, 1979b).

Denial

Denial is a normal way to protect oneself, maintain hope, emphasize the favorable, and minimize the unfavorable at a time of trauma. Parents may even delay taking the child to a physician in an attempt to avoid unpleasantness or to deny reality. In a healthy adjustment, tragedy is accepted after initial denial, and a period of mourning is experienced. Denial can also take the form of "doctor shopping"; the parents want someone to say the diagnosis is incorrect (Vernon, 1979b).

Guilt

A feeling of some responsibility and guilt is an inevitable part of every parent's reaction to the discovery that the child has a problem. Perhaps the pregnancy was not wanted, or prenatal care was poor. The parents may feel that they are being "punished" for past sins or negative feelings about the pregnancy. Guilt should be recognized and resolved as part of the counseling process.

Blame

When a birth defect occurs, the disappointment and helpless frustration of having a handicapped child may be transferred to others. The physician who delivered the child or provided the prenatal care is a common target. It is also common for parents to blame each other or various relatives who may have a similar defect (Vernon, 1979b).

Helping Parents Adapt to the Affected Child

Genetic counselors must be sensitive to normal feelings and emotions and recognize them in parents of birth defective children. Clinicians also need to be aware of these feelings, which may last a day or a lifetime. The parents of a child who is receiving therapy may be experiencing a number of intense emotions for which the sensitive clinician can offer some guidance or referral for guidance.

Effective coping can begin when denial is replaced by acceptance of the diagnosis. Appropriate acceptance may also include realistic abandonment of hope for a total cure and normalcy. However, the physician may, out of misguided kindness, extend false hopes that research will come forth with a miraculous cure or that compensatory therapies will make the child normal. On the other hand, after the diagnosis has been accepted, the prognosis need not be hopelessly limited. For example, if the parents accept the fact that their baby is retarded, they can begin the necessary intervention programs. Even if the child is severely retarded, small gains can be triumphs. In many of the case histories in this book (cri du chat syndrome; Möbius syndrome; Crouzon syndrome; and femoral hypoplasia-unusual facies syndrome), individual children surpassed an original prognosis. An outstanding example of a parent who was realistic in her acceptance while striving for the best possible quality of life is the mother of the child with Hunter syndrome. Clinicians too can become involved in the process of effective coping; they can help parents to find the correct diagnosis, accept that diagnosis, and then set realistic goals for their child.

Self-help groups

The ideal time for parents to become involved with a self-help group is when they first find out that their child is handicapped. Most communities have many parent groups, including organizations of parents of mentally impaired children. Parents need to not only receive information but to be able to express grief and fear with others who understand their feelings (Vernon, 1979a).

THE GENETICS CLINIC

For the more common genetic disorders, an experienced physician may be an excellent genetic counselor. However, if there is a complicated problem, the expertise of a team approach in a genetics clinic may be warranted. Usually the family physician, pediatrician, or obstetrician will refer a patient to a genetics clinic, but the patient or parent may simply call the genetics clinic for an appointment. No referral source is generally required. The genetics clinic is a diagnostic and information clinic and does not give ongoing therapy or service. Patients may receive many follow-up contacts, but they usually visit the clinic just once. An essential service provided by the genetics clinic is referral to community agencies, such as mental health agencies, agencies for financial help and family planning, or intervention services for an affected child.

A book, *Clinical Genetic Service Centers*, listing university-based genetics centers as well as hospital-based, satellite, and other genetics units in the United States can be obtained from The National Clearinghouse for Human Genetic Diseases, 1776 East Jefferson Street, Rockville, MD 20852.

The March of Dimes publishes the *International Directory of Genetic Services*, which may be obtained from the Medical Education Division, March of Dimes Birth Defects Foundation, 1275 Mamaroneck Avenue, White Plains, NY 10605. Another agency that provides referral services to genetics centers is the National Genetics Foundation, Inc., 555 West 57th Street, New York, NY 10019.

The Role of the Clinician in the Genetics Clinic

Clinicians as genetics clinic staff

The genetics clinic staff commonly includes a physician, a genetic counselor, and a social worker as core participants. Speech-language clinicians are not usually a part of a genetics clinic staff. It is becoming commonplace to find a genetic counselor as part of a team where a clinician is also a member, such as an oral-cleft clinic. However, a clinician who is part of a genetics clinic staff can perform these same valuable services:

1. Provide information to other team members. Many children with birth defects exhibit language delay and hearing loss. Although the physician will routinely inquire about speech and language development, the clinician can provide comprehensive information about language and cognition. The Receptive Expressive Emergent Language Scale, REEL, (Bzoch & League, 1971) is a quick screening test that can be used in this situation. This test should be used only for initial screening and is not recommended for research data or as an in-depth diagnostic test.

2. Provide information to the parents. In a discussion with the parents of a Down syndrome child, for example, the clinician may provide information about the expectations for speech and language development in Down syndrome and precautions for prevention of conductive hearing loss. The clinician should inquire about the child's hearing status and provide the parents with information about the availability of hearing testing for their child. It should not be assumed that the family has sought out a support group. Information and phone numbers for self-help groups and early intervention programs in the community may be provided by the clinician. Other information included in this book concerning anticipated speech and language in various genetic disorders and effects of intervention may be used in counseling the parents.

3. Advocate intervention programs. The clinician who knows the importance of early intervention for maximum development must sometimes convince parents (and physicians) that the child's therapy should start as soon as possible. It may be necessary, with assistance from the social worker, to arrange transportation to appropriate therapies, or to instruct school personnel concerning special needs of children, such as those with tracheostomies and neural tube defects. It is important to follow up on suggestions for intervention and to be available for questions that the parents think of later. For the parent who wants literature on the child's disorder, the names of books on developmental disabilities and home programs (e.g., Hanson, 1977; Horstmeirer & MacDonald, 1978) can be provided by the clinician.

Clinicians as referral agents

There are three reasons for a clinician to consider patient referral to a genetics clinic or physician for genetic counseling: (a) The family needs accurate diagnosis. (b) The family needs accurate information, including risk of occurrence and prognosis. (c) The family needs help with coping with feelings and life situations that concern the disorder. Clinicians are prepared to deal with the speech and language effects of disorders and to help the families find other services. A number of parents of children with birth defects do not avail themselves of genetic follow-up services because they do not know how to enter the genetic service network. Others may be intimidated by an unknown system. Some parents may feel uncomfortable about seeking genetic services, fearing a possible stigma for having a gentic disorder in the family. Clinicians can be an invaluable referral source. They can locate the nearest genetics clinic, provide parents with the name and telephone number of the contact person, and offer an encouraging description of how the genetics clinic operates. Clinicians can explain to parents that diagnosis is the basis for prognosis and that understanding of the cause and nature of a child's problem is beneficial to the child. Reports of the visit to the genetics clinic are sent to the referral source, unless the parents ask that the information not be shared.

Referral may be not only appropriate but a legal necessity. The legal rights of unborn children stemming from a failure to provide genetic counseling have been discussed by many authors (Burt & Hecht, 1982; Greenfield, 1982; Lawrence, 1979) and will not be discussed here. However, clinicians should be aware of possible implications for the future of the profession from the case of Turpin v. Sortini (Audiology Update, 1983; "Who Pays," 1982) that involved audiology services. When the Turpin's first baby was born, she was tested by an audiologist, but it was not discovered that she was deaf. When the second child was born, she, too, failed to respond to sounds, and the diagnosis of deafness was made for both children. It was subsequently discovered that the Turpins were carriers of an autosomal recessive genetic deafness, and the parents sued the audiologist who had tested the first child on behalf of their second child. The California Supreme Court ruled that a child born with a hereditary affliction (deafness) can maintain a personal injury action against a health-care provider (audiologist) who negligently failed to advise the child's parents of the possibility of the hereditary condition before the child's conception and deprived them of the opportunity to choose not to conceive the child.

The implications of this decision for audiologists are far reaching. To protect themselves from further litigation, pediatric audiologists are advised by the American Speech-Language Hearing Association to refer all cases of diagnosed hearing impairment with unknown etiology to a genetic counselor, to expand at-risk criteria and procedures for screening, diagnosis, and management of infants (see Chapter 6), and to include a geneticist as an integral team member, as not only a viable option, but as a necessity (Audiology Update, 1983). The implication for clinicians as part of the health-care field is to be aware of the legal responsibility to refer patients for genetic counseling whenever it is appropriate.

REFERENCES

Abroms, K.I. Service delivery networks. In K.I. Abroms & J.W. Bennett (Eds.), *Issues in genetics and exceptional children* . San Francisco: Jossey-Bass, 1981.

Ad Hoc Committee on Genetic Counseling. Genetic counseling, *American Journal of Human Genetics*, 1975, *27*, 240-242.

Audiology Update. American Speech-Language Hearing Association, Professional Practices Division, Spring 1983, 9-10.

Burt, C.E., & Hecht, F. Tort liability in genetic diagnosis and genetic counseling. *Human Genetics*, 1982, 34:2, 353-355.

Bzoch, K.R., & League, R. *Receptive Expressive Emergent Language Scale.* Baltimore: University Park Press, 1971.

Golbus, M.S. The current scope of antenatal diagnosis. *Hospital Practice*, 1982, 17:4, 179-186.

Greenfield, V.R. Wrongful birth: What is the debate? *Journal of the American Medical Association*, 1982, 248:8, 926-927.

Hanson, M. *Teaching your Down's syndrome infant: A guide for parents.* Baltimore: University Park Press, 1977.

Horstmeier, D.S., & MacDonald, J.D. *Ready, set, go, talk to me.* Columbus, OH: Merrill, 1983.

Lawrence, S.V. Advances in genetics give rise to hosts of moral and legal problems. *Forum on Medicine*, 1979, 2:9, 588-589.

McCormack, M.K. Medical genetics and family practice. *American Family Physician*, 1979, 20(3), 142-154.

Milunsky, A. *Know your genes.* Boston: Houghton-Mifflin, 1977.

Milunsky, A. Prenatal diagnosis of genetic disorders. *American Journal of Medicine*, 1981, 70, 7-8.

Pernoll, M.L., King, C.R., & Prescott, G.H. Genetics for the clinical obstetrician-gynecologist. *Obstetrics and Gynecology Annual*, 1980, 9, 1-53.

Porter, I.H. In W. Stockton, *Altered destinies.* Garden City, NJ: Doubleday, 1979.

Standish, L. The loss of a baby. *Lancet*, 1982, *1*, 611-612.

Summer, G.K., & Shoaf, C.R. Developments in genetic and metabolic screening. *Family and Community Health*, 1982, 4:4, 13-29.

Vernon, McC. Counseling parents of birth-defective children. *Postgraduate Medicine*, 1979, 65:3, 197-200. (a)

Vernon, McC. Parental reactions to birth-defective children. *Postgraduate Medicine*, 1979, 65:2, 183-189. (b)

Weitz, R. The public, the primary physician and genetic counseling. *First Quarter*, 1981, 3:1, 13-16.

Who pays for a life not worth living? *Newsweek*, May 17, 1982, p.105.

8

Discussion of Research Needs in Birth Defects and Genetic Disorders

Throughout this book the need for research has been emphasized. Information that comes from other disciplines does not necessarily answer the professional questions of speech-language pathologists. The obvious barrier to genetic research by practicing clinicians is that the educational background of speech-language pathology is behavioral science, not laboratory science. It is evaluation of the communication behavior of children with genetic and environmental birth defects that is the unique expertise of the speech-language clinician. Research must address the variables of that behavior, which, in turn, can lead to the ultimate goals of treatment and prevention.

Research in Genetic Disorders

Research reports in this book on chromosomal and single-gene disorders have been descriptive, that is, a child or group of children known to have a disorder are identified; their cognition, speech, and language are described; and some generalizations concerning that behavior become apparent. Studies of a few children or even a single case study should not be discounted as inconsequential, but care must be taken to make these descriptive studies meaningful. Some basic principles for future research in this area may serve as guidelines:

1. Diagnosis of the disorder must be accurate. What is the birth defect or genetic disorder? Are there multiple anomalies? Multiple etiologies? The concept of heterogeneity, in which a number of possible genotypes may be responsible for a pheotype, must make

researchers suspicious of diagnoses. The diagnosis of a birth defect must be unquestionable if inferences about the speech and language of that birth defect are to be made. For chromosomal disorders, there should be confirmation from cytogenic studies. Pedigrees should be included in reports of single-gene and multifactorial disorders.

2. Clinicians will need to collaborate. Clinicians must be prepared to conduct interdisciplinary, collaborative research. We must rely on the expertise of physicians, biochemists, genetic counselors, hospital staffs, and occupational therapists. An example of a model collaborative study is that of Witkop and Henry in 1963. The broad nature of the study included laboratory findings, genetic analyses, and pedigrees, along with complete descriptions of speech, language, and eating behavior. Collaborative studies, in which several clinicians pool their clinical data, may be the only possible way to investigate rare syndromes.

3. Beware of reliance on IQ tests. Most of the descriptive studies in this book have used IQ tests for data concerning verbal and nonverbal abilities. However, the full-scale IQ score may be quite meaningless in the disordered child. Most IQ tests reflect a great number of factors other than intelligence. A child's inability to perform well on certain sections of intelligence tests, or on the entire test, may not be due to mental retardation, but to a variety of problems, including sensory deficit, perceptual dysfunction, emotional disorder, sociocultural deprivation, and so forth. Examples of verbal-performance discrepancies as a result of perceptual, visual, and motor deficits were apparent in the studies of Duchenne muscular dystrophy (Karagan & Zellweger, 1978) and hydrocephalus in spina bifida (Dennis et al., 1981). Furthermore, the suggestion that children with birth defects who spend much of their lives in hospitals or restricted environments have characteristic language patterns (Noonan syndrome, cocktail party syndrome, Down syndrome) must also be taken into account in the interpretation of the tests.

4. Use standardized diagnostic speech and language tests. Descriptive data do not make the contribution to the profession that is possible with normative data. Some promising studies cited in this book are suspect because of the testing instruments used. Likewise, the same test should be used for all the subjects in the study. In the case of rare disorders in which only a few subjects could be found, as in partial trisomy 9p syndrome (Owens & Beatty-Desana, 1981), the age range was too great to use the same instrument. The study of Duchenne muscular dystrophy (Karagan

& Zellweger, 1978) was particularly strong in this regard, because subjects were chosen within a 5-year age range and with similar physical disability so that the same evaluation instrument could be used.

5. Describe and interpret the clinical picture of the prelinguistic, linguistic, and phonological development of the disorder. What effect does the defect have on the anatomy and function of the speech and associated structures? Is language delay consistent with general delay, or is there an expressive-receptive discrepancy? If inconsistencies exist, they are important. What are the strengths and weaknesses in cognitive function? What is the clinical presentation of retardation, if any? What behaviors differ from overall delayed development? What part do the factors of sensory deficit, perceptual dysfunction, emotional disorder, and sociocultural deprivation play?

Recent studies of Down syndrome children are notable because not only have language and phonological development been analyzed, but prelinguistic and pragmatic behavior, physical characteristics, and motor development have also been shown to affect the Down syndrome child's ability to communicate. The body of research concerning Down syndrome is perhaps the most complete of the genetic disorders, and reasonably so, as Down syndrome has been among the most common genetic disorders seen in the clinician's case load. The incidence of Down syndrome may decrease with the availability of amniocentesis, and other disorders may become more prevalent and, thus, more in need of study in the coming years.

Prenatal Environmental Birth Defects: Cause and Effect

It is extremely difficult to link cause and effect in those birth defects that have no genetic transmission. Perhaps the time will come when particular prenatal conditions will be shown to cause particular language deficits, and we can direct our efforts to prevention of disorders. However, there are four obvious difficulties in making conclusions of cause and effect:

1. The lapse of time between the prenatal cause and the evidence of delayed language development.

2. The difficulty in obtaining an accurate case history, including medical records. It is impossible for the mother of an affected baby to remember everything she ate, drank, did, and was exposed to during pregnancy.

3. The sociocultural environment of the child. Research data on the development of children with secondary growth failure are

confused by the socioeconomic status of the homes in which they are reared.

4. Differences in individual threshold of susceptibility to damage. Not everyone who is susceptible to a disorder develops the disorder. Who is susceptible? What environmental factors act upon the susceptible individual in order for the disorder to develop? It is possible that we are predisposed to believe that our environment is being poisoned by toxic waste, nuclear energy, herbicides, and radiation, and it is tempting to blame a popular villain or something for which a big corporation or the government can be made to pay.

It is important to not make hasty inferences and insist on sound scientific data. The research method of choice is to identify the high-risk infants prenatally or at birth and evaluate their speech and language at regular intervals. For example, the infants of diabetic mothers or of mothers who receive chemotherapy, anticonvulsants, or other drugs during pregnancy are groups that may be identified prenatally for evaluation.

Research Implications for Therapy

In the introduction to this book, the triad of clinical practice was discussed: diagnosis, prognosis, and treatment. As clinicians, we are concerned with prognosis and treatment, and it is in these two areas that existing reports are most often disappointing. It is also in these areas that reports from the medical literature are strikingly different from those of speech pathology: treatment is described and its effectiveness is evaluated. Readers of this book may have wished for more discussion of therapy methods for the disorders presented. The lack of information in the area of therapy is undeniable.

Case reports should not only describe speech and language behaviors but should also give prognostic information. Reports that therapy was not effective are as useful as those that report improvement, because prognosis is established. The comparison of two adults affected by fetal alcohol syndrome (Streissguth, Herman, & Smith, 1978) was especially interesting in that intellectual stimulation apparently did not affect intellectual progress. In progressive disorders, are some communicative functions impaired more quickly than others in the expected course of decline?

Communicative strengths and weaknesses are very valuable for therapy planning. It is important to make a distinction between behavioral characteristics that are amenable to change and behaviors that are directly associated with the disorder and perhaps cannot be changed. For example, the information that Down syndrome children have phonologic strengths in the development of stop plosives and learn best through visual cues can be utilized in therapy.

Through careful description and interpretation of collected case reports and empirical research, as well as controlled studies, speech-language pathology may not be left behind in the rapidly progressing area of genetic research.

REFERENCES

Dennis, M., Fitz, C.R., Netley, C.T., Sugar, J., Harwood-Nash, D.C.F., Hendrick, A.B., Hoffman, H.J., & Humphreys, R.P. The intelligence of hydrocephalic children. *Archives of Neurology*, 1981, *38*, 605-615.

Karagan, N.J., & Zellweger, H.U. Early verbal disability in children with Duchenne muscular dystrophy. *Developmental Medicine and Child Neurology*, 1978, *20*, 435-441.

Owens, A., & Beatty-Desana, J. Communication functioning in trisomy 9p. *Journal of Communication Disorders*, 1981, *14*, 113-122.

Streissguth, A.P., Herman, C.S., & Smith, D.W. Intelligence, behavior and dysmorphogenesis in the fetal alcohol syndrome: A report on 20 patients. *Journal of Pediatrics*, 1978, *92*(3), 363-367.

Witkop, C.J., & Henry, F.V. Sjogren-Larsson syndrome and histidinemia, hereditary biochemical diseases with defects of speech and oral functions. *Journal of Speech and Hearing Disorders*, 1963, *28*, 109-123.

Appendices

CASE HISTORY FORM

The case history for the child at risk for a congenital or perinatal birth defect with developmental delay should investigate the following factors. Positive responses should prompt closer questioning in that area.

Prenatal History

1. Health of the mother during pregnancy - diabetes, viral infections, toxemia, preeclampsia, eclampsia, high blood pressure, heart or kidney disease, anemia, thyroid disease, or other chronic disease.
2. Age of parents at the time of birth (mother younger than 18 or older than 35; father older than 55).
3. Number of previous children.
4. Drugs, radiation, medication or substances taken during pregnancy (includes alcohol and smoking).
5. Work-place exposures during pregnancy.

Perinatal History of the Child

1. Labor unusually fast or prolonged
2. Birth weight
3. Head circumference (unusually large or small)
4. Jaundice (hyperbilirubinemia)
5. Resuscitation (bag and mask for 1 minute)
6. Seizures
7. Tremor
8. Presentation: cesarean, head first, breech
9. Problems with placenta or umbilical cord
10. Low Apgar score. (Score of 7-10 — breathing adequately, crying, pinkish in color, and active; 4-6 — may need some oxygen to assist in respiration, may need to have thick mucous suctioned from the throat; Less than 4 — may be limp, unresponsive, pale, usually not breathing; must have throat suctioned and help with breathing for several minutes (Apgar & Beck, 1972).

Postnatal History of the Child

1. Feeding difficulties
2. Length of stay in hospital
3. Weight gain. Weight should double the birth weight at 4 months, triple by 12 months. (See growth charts.)
4. Height increase. In general, height should increase by 10 in. by 12 months and double the birth height by 4 years.
5. Head circumference. In general, should increase by 10 in. by 12 months.
6. Motor milestones: age child sat, walked, drank from a cup.
7. Signs of dysmorphology (See Chapter 1).

EVALUATION

A comprehensive assessment should have two parts: (a) reflexes and oromusculature and (b) cognitive function, including speech and language. The comprehensive assessment of choice is done by the clinician as part of an interdisciplinary team that also includes an occupational therapist and/or a physical therapist. The child's speech apparatus does not end with a distinct boundary somewhere around his lips or below his lungs. His whole body may be involved in the speech process and the members of the evaluation team should forget the usual arbitrary boundaries of their profession.

There are two comprehensive instruments for the detection of delays in development in young children. A test given by occupational therapists is the Bayley Scales of Infant Development (Bayley, 1969). It has been well standardized and includes items of motor development and reflexes as well as cognition and language development. A useful screening test for developmental problems is the Denver Developmental Screening Scale (Frankenburg, Fandal, & Dodds, 1970). The Denver Scale gives four different age levels for each test item, showing when 25, 50, 75, and 90% of children develop each skill. More diagnostic tests are indicated with consistent low performance. A sample of the language section of the scale is given below with ages for the 50th percentile of performance:

Laughs — 1 month
Turns toward a voice from behind — 5.6 months
Imitates speech sounds — 7 months
Says "dada" or "mama" to mean the parent — 10.1 months
Uses three words besides "mama" or "dada" — 12.8 months

Combines two different words to make a meaningful phrase (such as "want milk") but not a single-idea combination like "thank you" — 19.6 months.

Names a single picture: cat, apple, duck, dog — 20.3 months

Evaluation of Reflexes and Central Nervous System

There are no organs used exclusively for speech; all structures have primary functions for survival that have been modified for speech: the respiratory system for breathing, the laryngeal valve to protect the lungs, and the articulators for eating. It is reasonable that if those structures do not perform their primary function, they will be expected to have some difficulty in performing their secondary function (speech) as well.

The occupational therapist will evaluate the basic reflexes; the rooting and asymmetrical tonic neck reflexes should be present at birth and become integrated (disappear). Biting and sucking should appear appropriately. The absence of these reflexes, or the presence of reflexes that should have disappeared, denote an immature or damaged central nervous system. The presence of hypotonicity or hypertonicity in the musculature should be noted. (A child who has suffered asphyxia may have both.) The occupational therapist will also note the presence of marked tremor. Tremor can be a nonspecific response of the central nervous system in newborns after a difficult birth, or it may be part of various prenatal problems, such as hypoglycemia. Severe tremor in the history of the perinatal period should be regarded as significant if there are other signs of central nervous system involvement or signs of dysmorphology (Berger, Sharf, & Winter, 1975).

It might seem reasonable that referral to a neurologist is appropriate if there is suspicion of central nervous system damage, but that referral is only necessary in special circumstances. A neurologist may be essential during the newborn diagnostic period, but a child who is being followed by a pediatrician or family practice physician has a physician who is aware of his growth and development from birth. A specialist in the practice of neurology is essential only if the child is having seizures or if there is a change in behavior, such as a marked increase or decrease in activity level (Benjamins and Maltz, 1982; Ferry, 1981). Very sophisticated brain-scanning devices that are effective for detection of brain tumors and subdural hematomas are still not effective in the diagnosis of developmental disorders.

Oromuscular Evaluation

If an occupational therapist is not available, the speech-language pathologist should ask about the child's feeding history and observe the child feeding to note hypotonicity or hypertonicity (Jones, 1982). In the following guide for questions and observations, the age in parenthesis is the average age for development/extinction of the behavior.

1. Is drooling noted in crawling? (15 months)
2. Is drooling noted while using hands for feeding or play? (18 months)
3. Is drooling noted during speech with two- or three-word combinations? (24 months)
4. Observe the child bring a cracker to his mouth. Is he able to bite through? (12 months). Hypotonic children may lack this strength and "munch" the cracker in a straight up-and-down fashion.
5. Does he move the cracker around in his mouth using the tongue for side-to-side action? (24 months)
6. Are the lips closed during the chewing or are they hypotonic? (21 months)
7. Does the tongue protrude during the swallow? (18 to 24 months)
8. Is there true rotary action of the jaw during the chewing? (24 months)
9. When drinking from a cup, does the jaw stabilize on the cup? (15 months)

Cognition and Language Evaluation

For speech-language testing alone, the Sequenced Inventory of Communication Development, SICD, (Hedrick, Prather, & Tobin, 1975) for ages 4 months to 4 years is recommended as a diagnostic, standardized test, which is part parent interview and part child performance. Receptive items of awareness, discrimination, and understanding, and expressive items of imitation, initiating, responsiveness, and verbal output are evaluated. A disadvantage is that the SICD yields scores only at 4-month age increments (4 months, 8 months, 12 months, 16 months, and 20 months, etc.). A child tested at a chronological age of 18 months must be given a score of either 16 months or 20 months. The Receptive Expressive Emergent Language Scale, REEL, (Bzoch & League, 1971) gives age levels of expressive and receptive language development by 1-month increments in the 1st year and 2-month increments from 12 to 36 months. The REEL can give descriptive data about a child's language development from a parent interview in a relatively short time. It should not be relied upon for normative data.

The clinician should note, in particular, discrepancies between any area of cognitive or language development and the child's overall development from the Bayley Scales or Denver Developmental Screening Scale. It is commonly assumed that expressive language cannot be better than receptive language. This may not be true in those cases of children who have severe physical disabilities, are verbose, and appear to have good vocabularies. Their language patterns may, in fact, be severely aberrant. The clinician should also note factors that might interfere with testing, that is, physical handicap, sensory deficit, perceptual dysfunction, emotional disorder, and sociocultural deprivation.

Referral for Diagnosis

Even the clinician with long experience must resist the urge to become a medical diagnostician. Labeling a child with a particular syndrome is obviously dangerous and can lead to emotional, if not legal, consequences. After a careful history has been taken and a speech-language or interdisciplinary evaluation done, if it appears that the child may have dysmorphology, the clinician must refer a patient to the proper professional for diagnosis. Chromosomal study is indicated for any child with mental retardation and evidence of dysmorphology for which the etiology is uncertain (Warkany, 1981). The two major resources for the clinician are the child's physician and the genetics clinic. The physician can provide karyotyping and is also the most appropriate referral for cerebral palsy as a result of perinatal injury. If the physician is not comfortable with dysmorphology, and/or other counseling is desired by the parents, the genetics clinic is an appropriate referral.

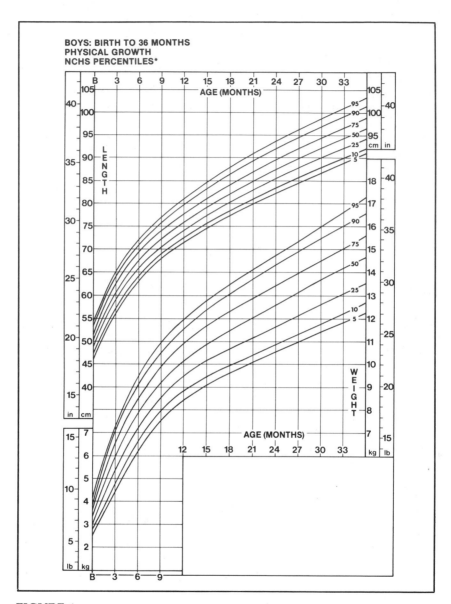

FIGURE 1.
Adapted from "Physical Growth: National Center for Health Statistics percentiles" by P.V.V. Hamill, T.A. Drizd, C.L. Johnson, R.B. Reed, A.F. Roche, W.M. Moore, 1979, *American Journal of Clinical Nutrition, 32,* 607-629. Data from the Fels Research Institute, Wright State University School of Medicine, Yellow Springs, OH. Courtesy of Ross Laboratories, Columbus, OH.

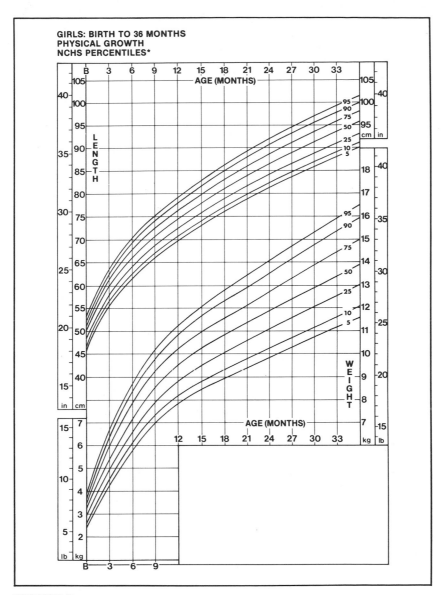

FIGURE 2.
Adapted from "Physical Growth: National Center for Health Statistics percentiles" by P.V.V. Hamill, T.A. Drizd, C.L. Johnson, R.B. Reed, A.F. Roche, W.M. Moore, 1979, *American Journal of Clinical Nutrition, 32,* 607-629. Data from the Fels Research Institute, Wright State University School of Medicine, Yellow Springs, OH. Courtesy of Ross Laboratories, Columbus, OH.

Glossary of Genetic Terms

Allele:

Alternative form of a gene at a given locus. For each autosomal locus, a person has two genes, which are either distinct from each other (allelic) or identical to each other (homozygous).

Autosomal:

Non-sex-linked; said of a gene carried on an autosome and therefore capable of being transmitted to either sex from either sex.

Carrier:

Heterozygote for a recessive disorder, whether autosomal or X-linked; a person or cell with one mutant recessive gene in the presence of a normal gene at a given locus.

Codominant:

Alleles are said to be codominant if both are equally detectable and their effects are additive.

Concordance:

Usually used in reference to twins, to indicate that both have a given trait. Discordance is the antithetical term.

Congenital:

Present at birth. No necessary connotation as to genetic or nongenetic causation.

Consanguinity:

Inbreeding.

Dizygotic:

Refers to twins derived from separate eggs (fraternal twins).

DNA:

Deoxyribonucleic acid, the genetic material of all cells; located within the chromosomes.

Dominant:	A mutant gene is said to be dominant when its expression overshadows or masks the normal allele. A disorder due to a dominant gene will be transmitted with a 50% likelihood if the other parent's genes are normal.
Empiric risk:	Risk estimates derived by actually sampling at-risk populations; for example, in the presence of an otherwise negative family history, the recurrence risk among first-degree relatives of a child with a neural tube defect is said to be 3 to 5%, because among 100 similar families, 3 to 5 will show an affected first-degree relative.
Enzyme:	A protein capable of carrying out a specific chemical reaction.
Expressivity:	The variability in severity of a genetic trait.
First-degree relative:	A person's first-degree relatives share 50% of his/her genes, and include parents, siblings, and offspring. Second-degree relatives share 25% of genes (e.g., grandparents, uncles, nieces, etc). Third-degree relatives share 12.5% of genes (e.g., first cousins, etc.)
Gene:	The unit of genetic function. The unit of genetic organization responsible for the constancy of a property or phenomenon from one generation, or one person, to another. Ultimately defined in chemical terms (one gene codes for one polypeptide) or in terms of the absence of crossing over between alleles.
Genotype:	The actual genetic makeup of an individual or cell, either with regard to a general, but defined, set of considerations (e.g., lipid metabolism, etc.), or with regard to a specific locus (e.g., blood groups). This concept underlies the notion that more than one combination of genes may correspond to a given phenotype.
Heterozygous:	Possessing different alleles at a given locus.

Homologous chromosomes:	Chromosomes that are alike, or very similar, in appearance and contain genes governing the same trait. Members of a pair of chromosomes.
Homozygous:	A person or cell is said to be homozygous for a given genetic locus when both alleles are identical.
Incest:	Consanguinity involving a mating between first-degree relatives (brother-sister, mother-son, or father-daughter) or between second-degree relatives.
Karyotype:	The chromosome constitution of an individual.
Locus:	The actual location of a gene along the length of a chromosome. This term applies whether or not the specific chromosome involved can be designated.
Lyon hypothesis:	The genetic inactivation of all X chromosomes in excess of one.
Meiosis:	The final sequence of cell divisions whereby germ cells are formed. In the penultimate division (meiosis I) the homologs of a pair are separated from each other (reduction division). In the final division (meiosis II) the chromatids for each homolog separate from each other. The resulting egg or sperm has the haploid number of chromosomes (23). Crossing over occurs in meiosis I (compare *Mitosis*).
Mendelian:	Refers to genes and resultant traits or disorders being transmitted according to specific patterns as elucidated by Gregor Mendel; Mendelian disorders are also referred to as single-gene disorders.
Mitosis:	The process of cell division in somatic cells. Each daughter cell winds up with the same number of chromosomes as the parent cell (46) (compare *Meiosis*).

Mosaic:
: An individual with cells of differing chromosome constitutions.

Monozygotic:
: Refers to twins derived from one egg (identical twins).

Multifactorial:
: Determined by multiple genetic and nongenetic factors. Polygenic is the term used to describe multiple genetic factors.

Mutation:
: A change in a gene's expression and chemical makeup.

Pedigree:
: The stylized, graphic way of portraying a family history; family tree.

Penetrance:
: Whether or not a dominant mutation is expressed at all. If expressed, no matter how slightly, the gene is penetrant, and if not expressed, it is nonpenetrant.

Phenotype:
: The observable or measurable expression of a gene or genes.

Proband:
: The affected individual who first comes to attention and brings the family to study. (Propositus)

Protein:
: Large molecules composed of amino acids. Proteins serve as enzymes or as structural components, such as hair, cartilage, or muscle fibers.

Recessive:
: The attribute of a trait that is expressed only when the responsible gene is present in homozygous state, or "double dose."

Sex-linked:
: A gene carried on a sex chromosome is sex-linked. Most often this term implies X-linkage, since there is only a very small number of specifiable genes on the Y-chromosome.

Sibs, siblings:
: Brothers and sisters.

Translocation: An exchange of pieces between nonhomologous chromosomes.

Trisomy: The presence of three homologous chromosomes instead of two.

REFERENCES

Apgar, V., & Beck. J. *Is my baby alright?* New York: Trident Press, 1972.

Bayley, N. *The Bayley Scales of Infant Development*. New York: The Psychological Corp., 1969.

Benjamins, D., & Maltz, A. *Psychological and neurological evaluation of children with speech and language disorders*. Paper presented to the Michigan Speech Language Hearing Association, Sugar Loaf, MI, March 20, 1982.

Berger, A., Sharf, B., & Winter, S.T. Pronounced tremors in newborn infants: Their meaning and prognostic significance. *Clinical Pediatrics*, 1975, *14*(9), 834-835.

Bzoch, K.R., & League, R. *Receptive-Expressive Emergent Language Scale*. Baltimore: University Park Press, 1971.

Ferry, P. *The developing brain and child language: Perspective of a pediatric neurologist*. Paper presented at the Workshop for Michigan Speech Pathologists in Clinical Practice, Detroit, December 5, 1981.

Frankenburg, W.K., Fandal, A.W., & Dodds, J.B. *Denver Developmental Screening Test*. Denver: Ladoca Publication Foundation, 1970.

Hamill, P.V.V., Drizd, T.A., Johnson, C.L., Reed, R.B., Roche, A.F., & Moore, W.M. Physical growth: National Center for Health Statistics percentiles. *American Journal of Clinical Nutrition*, 1979, *32*, 607-629.

Hedrick, D.L., Prather, E.M., & Tobin, A.R. *Sequenced Inventory of Communication Development*. Seattle: University of Washington Press, 1975.

Jones, J.L. *Assessment of oral-motor and pre-speech skills*. Paper presented at Western Michigan University, Kalamazoo, MI, February, 1982.

Warkany, J. Various indicators of central nervous system malformations. In J. Warkany, R.J. Lemire, & M.M. Cohen (Eds.), *Mental retardation and congenital malformations of the central nervous system*. Chicago: Year Book Medical Publishers, 1981.

Author index

Subject index